Amy Spangler's
BREASTFEEDING
A Parent's Guide

Amy Spangler, B.S.N., M.N., I.B.C.L.C.

Contributors
Heather D. Barbour, R.D., "Eating for two"
Karen Kerkhoff Gromada, R.N., "Breastfeeding twins"
Winnie Kittiko, M.S.N., "Especially for fathers"
Dennis L. Spangler, M.D., "Breastfeeding the baby
with a family history of allergic disease"

Illustrations and Production
Abby Drue, Inc.

Sixth Edition

ISBN 0-9627450-9-X

Library of Congress Catalog Card Number: 90-63214

This book is dedicated
to my husband, Dennis, for his faith;
to my children, Matthew and Adam, for their love;
to my mother, Phyllis, for her patience;
and to my father, Elmer, for his humor.
You are my inspiration.

CONTENTS

Author's note: Throughout this book, in an effort to keep the text clear, and easy-to-read, the baby is referred to as "he" or "him" when a personal pronoun was necessary.

FOREWORD

Breastfeeding is the most precious gift a mother can give her baby. Breastfeeding has numerous advantages for both infant and mother. A woman preparing for childbirth needs to think about how she is going to feed her baby before the baby arrives. After a discussion with her obstetrician or midwife and, of course, with her partner, a woman needs some help and reinforcement about her decision as she continues to think about it. Amy Spangler's *Breastfeeding, A Parent's Guide* provides the information necessary to make a comfortable decision, thoroughly reviewing all the questions parents have. No woman is born knowing how to breastfeed, and it is not a reflex that develops; she must learn. Learning how to breastfeed is well-described in this parent's guide. It can be read and re-read when breastfeeding is underway. Amy Spangler has made it clear and simple with her illustrations and instructions. It is pleasant reading.

As breastfeeding is initiated, questions may arise about the infant, the breasts, the milk, or the mother. The author has anticipated these questions and provides clear, concise answers. The discussion about less common problems that may occur is extremely valuable. It helps the reader determine what to watch for and when to call either the mother's or the infant's physician.

The highly publicized problems with breastfeeding are extremely rare and have been traced back in each case to the mother's lack of information about simple problems and the failure to ask for help from her healthcare provider. This book will be a reliable guide for parents in recognizing problems early and seeking help appropriately.

The author is an experienced nurse and mother who knows all phases of the childbirth process. Furthermore, Amy Spangler is an educator and knows how to share information in a clear, concise, complete manner. This parent guide is an ideal source of information. Now in its sixth edition, it has been well-received by healthcare practitioners to supplement their patients' understanding of breastfeeding and provide an ongoing reference source about special situations. It is an excellent resource of both the art and the science of breastfeeding for parents.

Ruth A. Lawrence, M.D.
Professor of Pediatrics,
Obstetrics & Gynecology
University of Rochester
School of Medicine & Dentistry

In 1970, when I began teaching childbirth classes to new and expectant parents, fewer than 20% breastfed their babies. Today, an ever-increasing number choose to breastfeed. In an effort to provide parents with breastfeeding information and support, I began teaching a breastfeeding class in 1984. To encourage attendance, the classes were held once a month, in the evening and were provided free-of-charge. I knew that many expectant parents had never seen a mother breastfeed, so I invited breastfeeding mothers and fathers as well. I wanted parents to know that breastfeeding was easy. I wanted parents to know that breastfeeding was fun. I wanted parents to know that breastfeeding was flexible. I wanted parents to know that there were no rules or regulations.

In 1985, with the encouragement of the many parents I taught, I wrote the first edition of **BREASTFEEDING, A Parent's Guide**. It was published under the title, **A Practical Guide to Breastfeeding**. I understood that parents wanted a book that was clear, concise and easy-to-read, not a dictionary, not an encyclopedia, not a medical textbook but a simple yet complete guide to breastfeeding. Finally, after five editions, ten years and thousands of questions, I feel I have succeeded in producing that book. My sincere thanks to the hundreds of mothers and fathers who have allowed me to share in one of the most intimate experiences of their lives, breastfeeding their baby. I have learned as much from you as you have learned from me. I am forever grateful.

Amy Spangler

INTRODUCTION

One of the most important choices you will need to make as new parents is whether to breastfeed or bottle-feed your baby. While the benefits of breastfeeding for both mother and baby are quite clear, the choice to breastfeed, as well as breastfeeding success requires knowledge and support. A clear understanding of how the process works and knowledge of how to manage problems that may occur are helpful. However, encouragement and support seem to be the key to success.

Most physicians and parents agree that breastfeeding is the best method of infant feeding, yet many parents choose to bottle-feed their babies or stop breastfeeding after a brief period of time. Frequently their choice is based upon too little information, incorrect information or too little support. *Amy Spangler's BREASTFEEDING, A Parent's Guide* is a wonderful resource for breastfeeding parents. It is a practical step-by-step guide to breastfeeding. It deals honestly and directly with the advantages as well as the concerns. The review of milk production is simple yet complete and gives the reader a clear understanding of this natural process. The suggestions for beginning-to-breastfeed provide recommendations that can be changed to meet the needs of each mother and baby. The discussion of possible problems, special situations and common questions answers most of the concerns expressed by new parents.

The information found throughout this book, appropriate medical advice and encouragement and support from someone you trust will help those parents who choose to breastfeed, breastfeed successfully and encourage those who are undecided to seriously consider breastfeeding.

Richard Bucciarelli, M.D.
Professor of Pediatrics
Associate Chairman Department of Pediatrics
Chief of Division of Neonatology
University of Florida
Gainesville

ADVANTAGES OF BREASTFEEDING

 ## Advantages to Mother

Physical

- Women who breastfeed have less vaginal bleeding and less risk of hemorrhage (excessive bleeding) after birth. Breastfeeding (infant suckling) causes the release of oxytocin, a hormone produced in the body which makes the uterus contract.

- Uterine contractions caused by the oxytocin, limit the amount of vaginal bleeding and return the uterus to its non-pregnant size sooner.

- Milk production requires 500-1000 calories each day. One-half of the calories comes from the body fat mothers deposit during pregnancy. The remaining calories come from foods eaten each day. While many mothers lose unwanted pounds easily, high calorie foods with no nutritional value should be avoided.

- Breastfeeding may reduce the risk of breast cancer in young women.[1,2]

- Breastfeeding requires no mixing, no measuring and no clean-up making nighttime feedings quick and easy.

Social

- Breastmilk is inexpensive. It is always available and requires no sterilization or refrigeration.

- Breasts and babies are portable. Diapers are disposable. Travel is simple. With a little practice, mothers can breastfeed anywhere. Mothers who are shy or easily embarrassed might want to choose a quiet place where they will not be disturbed.

Emotional

- Breastfeeding promotes a special relationship between a mother and baby, a closeness that comes with time and touch, a bond that lasts forever.[3]

- Breastfeeding provides an opportunity for mothers to rest during the day, something every new mother needs.

- With one hand free, breastfeeding allows a mother to share her time and attention with other children or take care of personal needs.

Advantages to Baby

Physical

- Breastmilk is nutritionally perfect, human milk for human infants. Human milk changes to meet the needs of a growing baby, something formula cannot do.[4,5]

- Breastmilk contains important nutrients as well as special protective factors, nature's way of safeguarding the immature newborn against infections.[6,7,8] As a result, breastfed babies have fewer illnesses, fewer doctor visits and fewer hospitalizations.

- Breastfeeding lowers the risk of asthma, colic, food allergy and eczema in those infants with a family history of allergy.[9,10,11]

- Breastmilk is readily available and requires no preparation, sterilization or refrigeration. This is very important for mothers and infants in developing countries where food supplies are limited or spoil easily.

- Breastmilk may contain nutrients or other substances that promote nervous system development and affect intelligence.[12]

- Breastfeeding reduces the risk of Sudden Infant Death Syndrome (SIDS), the leading cause of death in infants after one month of age.[13,14,15] To further reduce the risk of SIDS:

    ✓ sleep your baby on his back only (do not sleep your baby on his tummy or his side)

    ✓ keep your baby comfortable (do not let your baby get too hot or too cold)

    ✓ keep your baby in a smokefree environment during pregnancy and the first year of life

Emotional

- Breastfeeding gives babies a chance to touch, to smell, to hear, to see, to taste, to know their mother from the first moment of birth.

Common Concerns

There are no disadvantages to breastfeeding. However, there are certain factors which some women may find bothersome. As a result, some mothers may choose to breastfeed for a shorter period of time. Remember, any amount of breastfeeding will benefit you and your baby.

• Breastfeeding may limit your freedom for the first 4-6 weeks while you are building a milk supply and learning to breastfeed. However, this gives you a chance to rest and get to know your baby.

• Leaking can be annoying in the early weeks when babies are feeding at irregular times, however, leaking is a good sign of milk production and milk release.

• Breast nipples may be tender in the beginning when the baby first attaches to the breast. This is normal. However, do not confuse tenderness with pain. Breastfeeding should not be painful if the baby is positioned correctly on the breast.

• The quantity of milk taken at each feeding cannot be measured. However, frequent, watery stools will let you know that your baby is getting enough to eat.

• Breastmilk is easily digested producing loose, frequent, watery stools. However, there is little or no odor.

• Because breastmilk is easily digested, breastfed babies may feed more often and may not sleep through the night for several weeks or months. However, the same is true of many formula-fed babies. When your baby is 6-12 weeks old you can begin to lengthen the nighttime sleep period if necessary. You can delay nighttime feedings by diapering, walking and rocking.[18]

• You will need to limit your alcohol intake. However, you do not need to avoid certain foods unless they make your baby fussy or you have a family history of allergy.

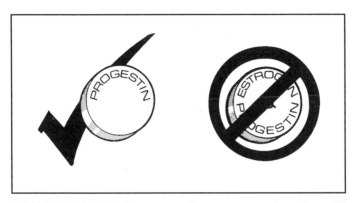

ILLUSTRATION 1: Breastfeeding mothers should avoid birth control pills that contain estrogen. Birth control pills that contain *progestin only,* are safe.

- Natural child spacing can be achieved with unrestricted, unsupplemented breastfeeding. However, breastfeeding schedules and routines that delay or decrease breastfeedings or include early introduction of non-breastmilk supplements may result in a return of fertility (ability to get pregnant). If pregnancy is not desired, birth control is suggested. Methods of birth control include birth control pills (progestin only), condom, diaphragm, IUD (intrauterine device), vaginal sponge, cervical cap, spermicidal cream, foam or jelly, Norplant (implant) and Depo-Provera (injection). Birth control pills that contain estrogen and progestin (combination pills) are not recommended. Estrogen decreases breastmilk production and may affect growth and development of babies.[16] However, birth control pills that contain progestin only are safe and may be taken by breastfeeding mothers (Illustration 1).[17]

UNDERSTANDING MILK PRODUCTION

Anatomy of the Human Breast

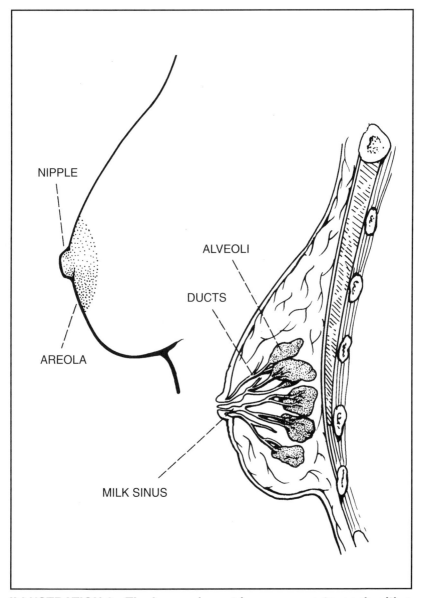

ILLUSTRATION 2: The human breast has many parts, each with a special function.

To increase your enjoyment of breastfeeding, a basic understanding of how the breast functions during lactation (milk production) may be helpful (Illustration 2).

To nourish a baby at the breast two things must happen (1) milk production and (2) milk release.

Milk Production: Milk production takes place in the alveoli, grapelike clusters of cells located inside the breast. Infant suckling or breastfeeding is the stimulus for milk production and should begin as soon after birth as possible. The amount of milk produced is determined by the amount of breastfeeding which takes place. Early, frequent feedings, 8-12 breastfeedings in a 24-hour period, will usually produce a good supply of milk.

Factors which influence milk production include number and length of breastfeedings and position of the baby on the breast. To increase your milk supply:

• Position the baby correctly on the breast. When positioned correctly his tongue should be over his lower gum, between his lower lip and the breast. His lips should turn out, like a fish, and lie flat against the breast. His chin should press firmly into the breast. His nose should gently touch the breast (Illustration 12).[19]

• Breastfeed at least every 2-3 hours during the day (6am- 12am). Time from the beginning of one feeding to the beginning of the next.

• Breastfeed as long as the baby wishes on the first breast before offering the second breast. Watch your baby, not the clock. When the baby stops suckling or falls asleep at the first breast, break the suction, burp him, wake him and offer the second breast. If the baby breastfeeds poorly on the first breast, put him back on the first breast. Breastfeed well on one breast before offering the second breast.

• Offer both breasts at every feeding, however do not be concerned if the baby seems satisfied with one breast. Each breast can provide a full meal. If necessary, pump or hand express to relieve the fullness in the second breast.

• Begin each feeding on the breast offered last.

Milk Release: When the baby begins to breastfeed the following occur (Illustration 3):

• The suckling stimulates the nerves inside the nipple to send a message to the brain.

• The brain receives the message and signals the pituitary gland to release two hormones, prolactin and oxytocin.

• Prolactin causes the alveoli, the milk-producing cells in the breast, to make milk.

• Oxytocin causes the small muscles around the milk-producing cells to contract. Milk is squeezed out of the cells and down to the collecting pools or milk sinuses located beneath the areola, the dark part of the breast around the nipple. Correct positioning of the baby's mouth on the breast puts pressure on the milk sinuses, causing the milk to flow out through the openings in the nipple.

This sudden release of milk from the breast is called the let-down reflex or milk-ejection reflex. It may take several seconds or several minutes of suckling for this release of milk to occur. It may also take several days for this reflex to develop fully. Many mothers experience more than one let-down during each feeding. You may feel a tingling or burning sensation in the breasts when the milk lets-down or you may notice milk leaking from one breast while the baby is breastfeeding from the opposite breast. Don't be concerned if you observe nothing, every mother is different. Simply watch your baby. When your milk lets-down, his suckling pattern will change from short, rapid bursts of suckling to a slower, rhythmic, suckle-swallow pattern. The suckle-swallow pattern causes movement in the upper jaw which makes the baby look like he is wiggling his ears.

Oxytocin also causes the uterus to contract, resulting in "afterbirth pains." These contractions may be felt while breastfeeding for several days after birth. Though uncomfortable, they limit vaginal bleeding and help the uterus return to its non-pregnant size.

Factors which can affect milk release include:

• embarrassment	• pain
• lack of confidence	• stress
• lack of encouragement and support	• tiredness

22

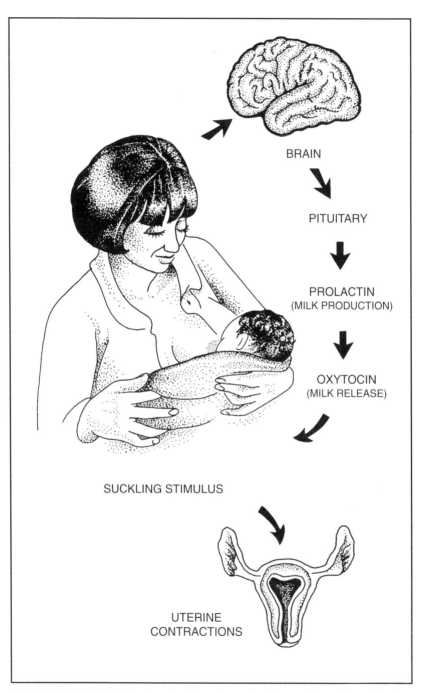

BRAIN

PITUITARY

PROLACTIN
(MILK PRODUCTION)

OXYTOCIN
(MILK RELEASE)

SUCKLING STIMULUS

UTERINE
CONTRACTIONS

ILLUSTRATION 3: Understanding how the breast functions during milk production and milk release can make breastfeeding easier.

Milk Composition

There are three types of human milk: colostrum, transitional milk and mature milk. Although each contain similar nutrients, they vary in content. From 0-5 days after birth, colostrum is produced; from 5-15 days transitional milk is produced; after 15 days mature milk is produced. This change is gradual and may occur unnoticed. The rate of change will vary depending upon which pregnancy this is for the mother.

Lactation, the period of milk production, begins with the appearance of colostrum. Colostrum is a clear or yellowish fluid. It is high in protein, low in fat and rich in antibodies which protect infants from infection. Colostrum is a natural laxative which helps to remove meconium from the lower bowel of newborns. Meconium is a thick, black, tarry substance that contains bilirubin. When bilirubin increases, jaundice occurs. Early passage of meconium decreases jaundice in the newborn.

The content of transitional milk changes gradually over a 10-15 day period. While sugar, fat and calories increase, protein and antibodies decrease, until the levels of mature milk are reached.

Mature milk has two parts, hindmilk and foremilk. Foremilk or "first milk" collects in the milk sinuses (Illustration 2). Foremilk is high in protein, low in fat and low in calories, giving it a thin, watery appearance. Hindmilk or "behind milk" collects in the milk-producing cells or alveoli. Hindmilk is high in protein, high in fat and high in calories, giving it a thick, creamy look. Foremilk is obtained at the beginning of a feeding while hindmilk is obtained at the end of a feeding (Illustration 4).

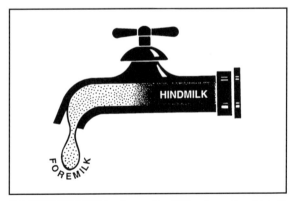

ILLUSTRATION 4: If you limit the length of each breastfeeding, babies get little or no hindmilk, which contains the fat babies need to grow.

Hindmilk contains the calories necessary for the rapid growth of newborns. When breastfeeding routines limit the length of feedings, babies do not get enough hindmilk or calories. To prevent this, breastfeed as long as the baby wishes on the first breast before offering the second breast. When the baby stops suckling or falls asleep at the first breast, break the suction, burp him and offer the second breast. If he breastfeeds poorly on the first breast, put him back on the first breast before offering the second breast.

Prenatal Hand Expression

Removal of colostrum from the breasts during pregnancy is not recommended. Hand expression or any manner of pumping the breasts can produce a breast infection or uterine contractions. Because the uterine contractions can cause premature labor, any possible benefit of prenatal expression is outweighed by the likely risks.[20]

PREPARING THE BREASTS FOR NURSING

Frequently women worry that the size and shape of their breasts will affect their ability to produce milk. Fat deposits determine breast size and shape. While these deposits protect the milk-producing cells in your breast, they do not affect your ability to produce milk. However, nipple size and shape can affect the ease of breastfeeding.

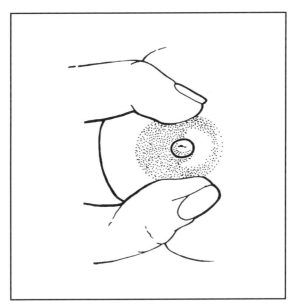

ILLUSTRATION 5: The pinch test will help you decide if your nipples are flat or inverted.

The Pinch Test (Illustration 5) will help you decide if your nipples are normal, flat or inverted (Illustration 6). Do the test on each nipple early in your pregnancy.

- Place your thumb and first finger at the base of the nipple near the edge of the areola.

- Press your thumb and first finger together.

- A normal nipple will protrude or come out.

- A flat or inverted nipple will retract or sink in (truly inverted nipples are rare).

If you see little or no movement of the nipple when you do the pinch test, put ice on the nipple for a few seconds. A flat or inverted nipple will sink in. A normal nipple will come out.

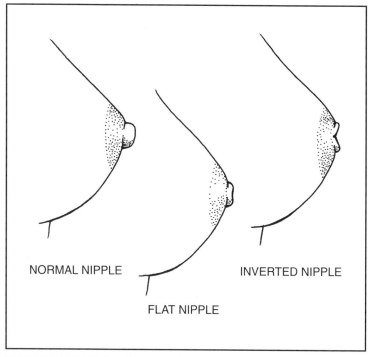

NORMAL NIPPLE

INVERTED NIPPLE

FLAT NIPPLE

ILLUSTRATION 6: Breast nipples come in all shapes and sizes and can affect the ease of breastfeeding.

Flat or Inverted Nipple Treatment

You can treat flat or inverted nipples with a breast shell, a two-piece glass or plastic device (do not use a rubber shield) which applies constant, even pressure to the areola, forcing the nipple to protrude through the center opening in the shell (Illustration 7). During the last weeks or months of your pregnancy, begin by wearing the shells for an hour or two each day. A snug bra will keep the shells in place. Slowly increase the time until the shells are worn 4-6 hours a day. To keep moisture from damaging the nipples, remove the shells every 2-3 hours and let the breasts air dry.[21]

27

Some women find the shells uncomfortable or embarrassing and prefer to wait until after birth to see if "latch-on" is difficult.[22] If the baby has difficulty latching on, a breast pump can be used before each breastfeeding to gently pull the nipple out. You can make a small, inexpensive pump using a peridontal syringe. Cut off the tip, reverse the barrel and insert the plunger (Illustration 8). Center your nipple inside the barrel and position the barrel against your breast. Apply gentle suction with the plunger for several seconds, release the plunger and repeat the suction until the nipple protrudes or comes out. Remove the syringe and quickly put the baby on the breast (See "Beginning to Breastfeed," p. 32).

While many books recommend nipple exercises or other forms of nipple preparation, nipple exercises or any form of nipple stimulation may produce uterine contractions and preterm labor. Therefore, both the benefits and the risks must be carefully considered. Nipple exercises (nipple pulling and rolling) or other forms of nipple preparation (rubbing the nipples with a towel or washcloth) do not prevent tender, painful nipples in the early weeks of breastfeeding.[23] Correct positioning of the baby on the breast seems to be the important factor affecting nipple pain.[24]

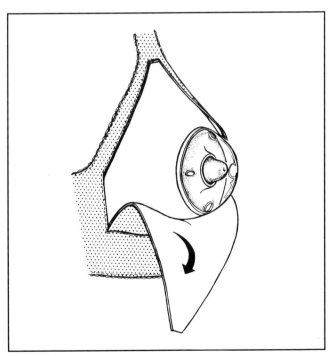

ILLUSTRATION 7: Breast shells can be used during pregnancy to correct flat or inverted nipples.

28

Women who plan to breastfeed but who are uncomfortable handling their breasts, might want to follow the simple suggestions for Prenatal Breast and Nipple Care, p.30.

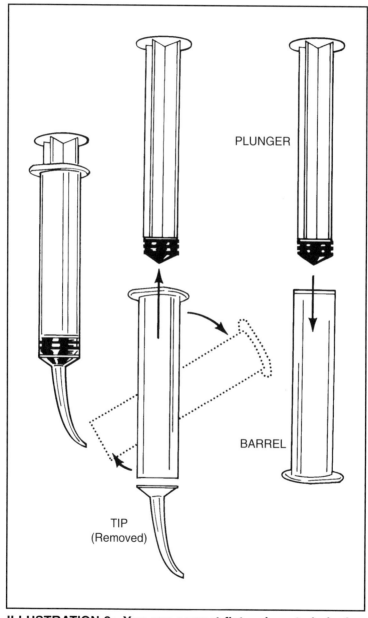

PLUNGER

BARREL

TIP
(Removed)

ILLUSTRATION 8: You can correct flat or inverted nipples using a small pump made from a peridontal syringe.

PRENATAL AND POSTPARTUM BREAST AND NIPPLE CARE

Prenatal Breast and Nipple Care

- The Glands of Montgomery, small pimple-like bumps in the areola, the dark part of the breast around the nipple, release an oily material which helps to keep the nipples clean and moist.

- If your nipple(s) are very dry, an unscented cream or lotion may be used. Use only a small amount, a little bit goes a long way.

- Expose your breasts to air and sunlight each day if possible. Be careful to avoid sunburn.

- Remove your bra for a period of time each day and allow your clothing to gently rub against the nipples. If you prefer, wear a nursing bra and release the flaps or cut a small hole in the center of a regular bra.*

*You do not need to wear a bra while you are pregnant or breastfeeding. However, if you prefer to wear a bra, you may find a nursing bra handy. For a proper fit, wait until the last weeks of your pregnancy. Choose a comfortable bra with a cotton cup, an adjustable strap and a simple flap-fastener. Avoid bras with underwires or bras that are too tight or bind, making it difficult to remove milk from all parts of the breast. Remember to remove your bra at bedtime, unless you are leaking and need to wear nursing pads.

Postpartum Breast and Nipple Care

- Use only clear water when you wash your breasts. Wash infrequently to avoid unnecessary drying.

- Avoid the use of soaps, creams, lotions and ointments.

- Whenever possible, air dry your nipples after each breastfeeding.

- Change nursing pads frequently. Do not use pads with plastic liners.

- If your nipple(s) get tender, put a few drops of breastmilk or colostrum on the areola and nipple after each breastfeeding, until the tenderness improves.

- If your nipple(s) become cracked or bleed, put a small amount of modified lanolin* on the tender area after each breastfeeding to aid healing.[25]

*Modified lanolin, Lansinoh, is a purified form of lanolin. It contains less pesticide residue and free lanolin alcohol than other lanolin products, making it safe for mothers and babies.

Beginning to Breastfeed

Step-By-Step Suggestions

1. Breastfeed as soon as possible after birth, if the condition of mother and baby permits.

2. Choose a comfortable position (Illustrations 9 & 10). Place the baby on his side facing your breast, at the level of your chest. If necessary, use pillows to support the baby.

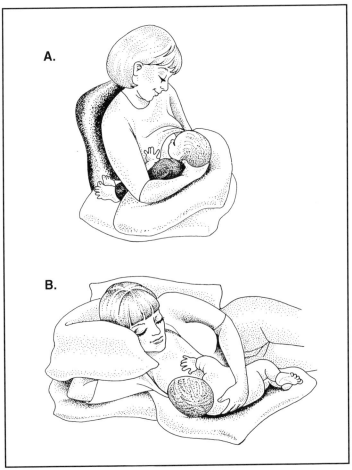

ILLUSTRATION 9: Choose a breastfeeding position that is comfortable, (A) Football, (B) Sidelying.

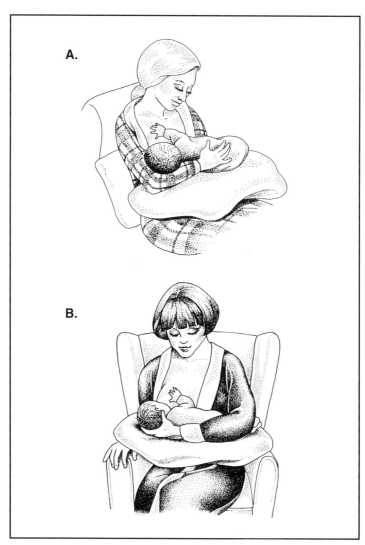

ILLUSTRATION 10: Use different breastfeeding positions each day, (A) Cradle, (B) Modified Football.

3. Using a "C" hold cup the breast in your hand. Place your fingers below the breast and your thumb above (Illustration 11A). Women with a large hand and a small breast may prefer the "scissors" hold (Illustration 11B).[26] If you choose this hold, be careful to place your fingers outside the areola. When your baby is positioned correctly on the breast, much or all of the areola may disappear. However, this will depend upon the size of your areola and the size of your baby's mouth.

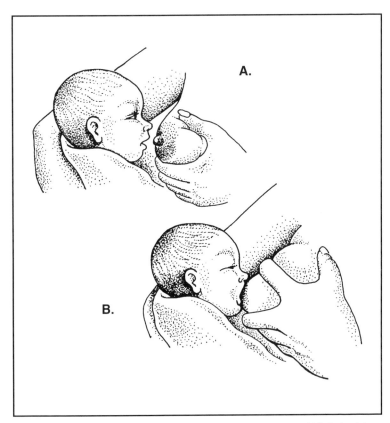

ILLUSTRATION 11: Support your breast using a (A) C-hold or (B) Scissors hold. Remember to keep your thumb and fingers outside the areola.

4. If necessary, express a small amount of colostrum to soften the breast and permit correct positioning of the baby's mouth. This will also encourage the baby to attach or "latch on" if colostrum is easily obtained.

5. Using the baby's rooting reflex, gently rub the baby's cheek nearest your nipple. As he turns toward the breast, tickle his upper and lower lip with your nipple until his mouth opens wide.

6. Center your nipple in his open mouth and quickly bring him toward the breast. Do not lean forward. Bring the baby to you. When positioned correctly his tongue should be over his lower gum between his lower lip and the breast. His lips should turn out and lie

flat against the breast. His chin should press firmly into the breast. His nose should gently touch the breast (Illustration 12). Hold the baby close. This will prevent unnecessary pulling on the breast and keep the baby positioned correctly.

7. Babies breathe through their noses. Often the nose touches the breast when the baby nurses. If the nose is buried in the breast, you can lift up gently on the breast with your fingers below to let air enter the nose. Do not press down on the breast with your thumb above or your nipple may slip out of his mouth.

8. Do not watch the clock. Watch your baby. When he stops suckling or falls asleep at the first breast, break the suction, burp him and offer the second breast. If he breastfeeds poorly on the first breast, wake him and put him back on the first breast. If necessary pump or hand express to relieve fullness in the second breast. It is more important that he breastfeed well on one breast, getting foremilk and hindmilk, than that he breastfeed on both breasts.

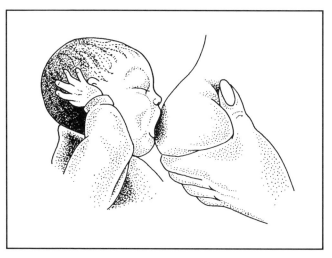

ILLUSTRATION 12: Position your baby correctly on the breast.

9. Break the suction by gently sliding your finger between the baby's gums to the end of the nipple or simply press the breast near his mouth making a small dimple with your finger (Illustration 13).

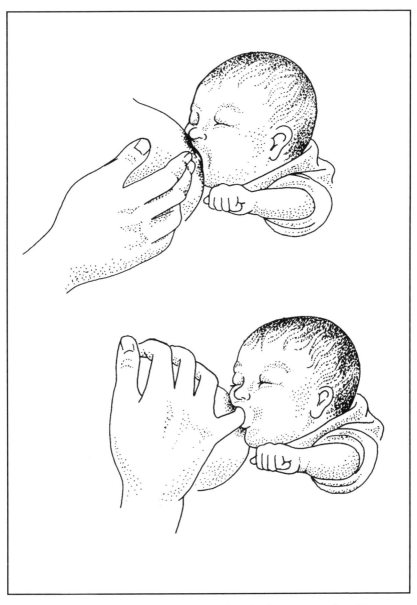

ILLUSTRATION 13: Break the suction before removing the baby from the breast.

10. Breastfeeding should not be painful if the baby is positioned correctly on the breast. You might feel tenderness when the baby first latches on. However, the tenderness should stop as he draws the nipple into his mouth. If the tenderness continues, remove the baby from the breast and try again.

11. Breastfeed on demand or request, whenever the baby seems fussy or hungry. Hungry, alert babies breastfeed well, which will increase your milk supply.[27] Expect to breastfeed every $1\frac{1}{2}$-3 hours during the day and every 2-3 hours at night. Occasionally a sleepy baby will not demand or ask to eat often enough. Therefore, during the first 2-4 weeks, if your baby does not actively wake or cry, you may need to watch for signs of lighter sleep such as sucking movements, sucking sounds or restlessness and offer the breast at those times. Additional suggestions for waking a sleepy baby include:

   • remove all blankets
   • change his diaper
   • wash his bottom with a cool washcloth
   • massage his feet
   • place him in your lap in a sitting position, support his chin in one hand, massage his back with the other hand

12. Breastfeed as long as the baby wishes on the first breast before offering the second breast.[28] When he seems satisfied or falls asleep at the first breast, break the suction, burp him and offer the second breast. This will help to build a better milk supply and prevent breast fullness. Do not be concerned if the baby seems satisfied with one breast. Each breast can provide a full meal. If necessary, pump or hand express to relieve fullness in the second breast.

13. Offer both breasts at each feeding. Begin each feeding on the breast offered last.

14. Support your baby well in whatever breastfeeding position you choose (Illustrations 9 & 10). This will prevent unnecessary pulling on the breast, keep the baby positioned correctly and lessen nipple tenderness.

15. Have fun and relax!

CONTINUING TO BREASTFEED

The early weeks are a learning experience for the entire family, so relax and enjoy this time together. While a new mother can take care of herself and her baby, she should leave the household chores to others, cobwebs can wait! Nap at least once a day when the baby naps. The frustrations of parenting seem greater when parents are exhausted from too little sleep. If necessary, limit visits and visitors. Continue to eat a balanced diet and drink to satisfy your thirst (6-8 glasses a day).

As soon as your baby is breastfeeding well and gaining weight, about 4 weeks after birth, you can begin to let him set his own feeding schedule. Remember, every baby is different. Some babies continue to breastfeed every 2-3 hours during the day and night, for many weeks or months. Other babies breastfeed every 1-2 hours when awake and sleep for longer periods of time. You may need to express a small amount of breastmilk while your baby is sleeping to relieve fullness. Express only enough milk to relieve fullness and prevent engorgement. Do not express so much milk that you tell the breasts to keep making the same amount. Within 24-48 hours, your breasts will respond to the change in demand and make less milk.

You can begin light exercise 2-4 weeks after birth. However, listen to what your body tells you. Many mothers eager to resume their active lifestyle do too much too soon and quickly regret it.

EATING FOR TWO

There are many questions that mothers have concerning nutrition during breastfeeding. How many calories should I eat while breastfeeding? How can I lose the extra weight I gained during my pregnancy? Are vitamin and mineral supplements necessary?

Nutritional needs vary with how much milk is produced. For example, the woman who supplements her baby with formula, in addition to breastfeeding, does not need as many calories as the woman who breastfeeds twins. It is often recommended that a woman eat 500 additional calories daily while she is breastfeeding. However, most women can produce enough milk while eating about the same number of calories as they did before they were pregnant. For example, a woman whose pre-pregnancy weight was 125 pounds, probably needs about 1800 calories while she is breastfeeding. This way some of the calories needed to make the breastmilk are taken from fat stored during pregnancy.

Most women find they lose excess weight gained during pregnancy over a six-month period. Although this may seem a slow rate of weight loss, restricting calories to lose weight more quickly is not recommended, since it can interfere with milk production. Although it can be argued that even malnourished mothers produce high quality milk, it is at the expense of their own health. For example, if the mother does not eat enough calcium, her bones will be used as a source of calcium and will become weakened as a result. By eating enough calories, you can be certain that other nutrient needs are met as well, including those for protein, vitamins and minerals.

A balanced breastfeeding diet includes extra servings of protein and calcium. Foods such as citrus fruits, vegetable oils and green, leafy vegetables are also slightly increased over the normal diet, to meet additional needs for vitamins C, E and folic acid. Although it is important to drink water and other fluids whenever you are thirsty, there are no strict fluid requirements while you are breastfeeding.

As long as the mother eats a balanced diet, the only supplement she may need while breastfeeding is iron. Extra iron is helpful in replacing the iron stores lost during pregnancy. Frequently, mothers choose to continue their prenatal vitamins while they are breastfeeding.

Individuals who are unable to eat one or more of the major food groups must plan their diets more carefully. This may be the case when a woman does not tolerate milk. Calcium needs can still be met by eating several servings of dark, green, leafy vegetables each day or by taking a calcium supplement. A vegetarian diet is not a problem as long as some animal protein such as eggs or milk products is included in the diet. Women who follow a strict vegetarian diet which does not include animal protein must choose foods carefully to obtain enough calories and protein. They may also need to take vitamin B^{12} and calcium supplements to meet their own needs as well as those for milk production.

Suggested Breastfeeding Diet

Food Groups	Number of Servings	Examples of One Serving
MILK/MILK PRODUCTS	3-4*	1 cup milk 1 cup yogurt $1^1/_2$ cups cottage cheese $1^1/_2$ ounces cheese $1^1/_2$ cups ice cream
MEAT/MEAT SUBSTITUTES	2-3	2 ounce lean meat, fish, poultry 1 egg 1/2 cup cooked beans 2 Tbsp. peanut butter 1 ounce cheese 1/2 cup tuna 1/2 cup nuts or seeds
CEREAL, BREAD PASTA, RICE	6-8	1 slice bread 1/2 roll, muffin, biscuit 1 tortilla 1/2 cup hot cereal 3/4 cup cold cereal 1/2 cup rice, noodles, pasta
FRUIT/VEGETABLE **Vitamin C**	5-7 1	1/2 cup juice 1 medium orange 1/2 grapefruit 3/4 cup cooked broccoli, bell pepper, cabbage
Vitamin A	1	1 cup raw or 1/2 cup cooked spinach, broccoli, brussel sprouts, greens, romaine lettuce 1/2 cup apricots 1 cup berries or melon
Others	3-5	1/2 cup fruit juice 1/4 cup dried fruit 1 fresh medium fruit 1/2 cup raw vegetables
FATS,OILS, SWEETS	Limited amounts	

*Occasionally, something in the mother's diet will make a baby fussy. Foods which frequently cause fussiness include milk products, eggs and nuts. If you have a family history of allergic disease or a very fussy baby you might want to limit these foods in your diet. In addition, avoid caffeine-containing foods such as coffee, tea, chocolate and many carbonated beverages.

41

ESPECIALLY FOR FATHERS

 As a new father you will experience many feelings and emotions. Adjusting to fatherhood takes time, so be patient. Try to relax and enjoy each moment because it doesn't get any easier than this.

Breastfeeding is the best choice for every baby and fathers benefit too! Happy, healthy babies need fewer doctor visits and fewer hospitalizations, making parenting easier. A breastfed baby, snug and content against your chest gives you confidence in your ability to care for your baby. Nighttime feedings are simple when there is no formula to mix, measure or warm. In addition, breastfed babies are portable, good news for active parents!

Breastfeeding is the natural way to feed your baby but it does not always come naturally. Sometimes a mother, father and baby know just what to do, more often they need to be taught. It will help to learn all that you can while you are pregnant (fathers are pregnant too)! This book will answer most of your questions, so be sure to read it carefully and keep it handy. Practice breastfeeding as often as you can while you are in the hospital. Keep the baby with you as much as possible and ask every question that comes to mind. Watch how the nurses help with breastfeeding and ask them to show you. Remember that mothers and babies need to breastfeed frequently and rest often. If necessary, limit the number of visitors and the length of visits. While some mothers are comfortable breastfeeding in front of family and friends (both male and female), many are not. It is important that a mother be relaxed. You know your partner best. So don't hesitate to speak up.

While it is nice to have help at home, family and friends can be a source of tension as well as a blessing if their knowledge of breastfeeding is limited. You may need to explain politely the benefits of breastfeeding, the importance of frequent feedings, feeding on demand and nighttime feedings. Explain that it's better for mother and baby to nap during the day and breastfeed at night, than for Grandma to bottle-feed the baby so mother can sleep through the night. Ask Grandma to take care of the home while your partner takes care of herself and the baby but remember to tell Grandma how much you appreciate her help as you learn to be a father to her grandchild.

Breastfeeding is an important part of parenting but equally important is the time you spend with your baby and the special moments you share. Find something that you enjoy doing with your baby and make it into a routine. Taking walks, splashing in the tub, listening to music, playing games or simply watching TV or reading the newspaper are ways for you and your baby to spend time together and get to know one another.

Many parents ask, "When will things get back to 'normal'?" The truth is, never! Your idea of "normal" will need to change. The two-seater sports car of your youth may no longer be practical and minivans may look more appealing. You will need to adjust priorities and establish goals for a life that now includes another person. There may be little time at first for individual needs, however, as you learn to be a father to your baby remember to be a friend and lover to your partner.

Despite all your efforts there will be times when things do not go well. Be prepared for the day when you arrive home from work to find your partner still in her nightgown. She and the baby are crying, the laundry needs to be done and there is no dinner. Perhaps your day was just as bad! Instead of becoming angry, put a load of clothes in the washer, take the baby for a walk (it will relax all of you), order a pizza for dinner and suggest that your partner make a cup of tea and take a warm bath. She will love you for understanding and it will keep you both from saying things you might later regret.

Parenting is never easy, so relax and enjoy this time with your baby. Fathering a breastfed baby is a special joy, the benefits of which last a lifetime.

Managing Possible Problems

Blisters

 Cause:

A blister may form on the nipple or areola of the breast. Blisters are caused by friction or pressure on the skin when the baby breastfeeds. Blisters are usually filled with clear fluid, but can be filled with blood. While the fluid can affect the taste of the milk, it will not hurt your baby. Because the fluid protects the new skin underneath, blisters should not be opened or drained. Leave them alone and they will heal.

 Recommended Treatment:

• To soften the blister and prevent cracking, put warm water on the blistered area using a towel or washcloth. Do this before each breastfeeding.

• Position the baby correctly on the breast (Illustration 12).

• Avoid those breastfeeding positions which put pressure on the blistered area.

• If necessary, begin each breastfeeding on the breast without the blister. When a let-down occurs switch to the breast with the blister.

• If necessary, limit breastfeeding time to 10-20 minutes on the breast with the blister and breastfeed more often, every $1\frac{1}{2}$-3 hours.

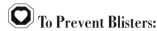 To Prevent Blisters:

• Position the baby correctly on the breast. Tickle his upper and lower lip with your nipple. When his mouth opens wide, center your nipple in his open mouth and quickly bring him toward the breast.

• Use 2-3 different breastfeeding positions each day.

• Hold the baby close and tight to prevent unnecessary pulling on the breast.

• Offer both breasts at every feeding. Do not be concerned if the baby seems satisfied with one breast. Begin each feeding on the breast offered last.

Breast Infection (Mastitis)

 Cause:

Bacteria can enter the breast through an opening in the nipple or a break in the skin. When breastfeedings are delayed or missed or when babies are feeding at irregular times the breasts overfill and a breast infection can occur. The mother has "flu-like" symptoms with fever. The breast is red, hot and painful.

 Recommended Treatment:

• Call your doctor. A prescription medication (antibiotic) may be necessary. Although your symptoms may improve in 24-48 hours, take the medication until it is gone (10-14 days).

• Continue to breastfeed on both breasts. The infection will not harm your baby. Breastfeed every $1\frac{1}{2}$-3 hours during the day and every 2-3 hours at night. Start each feeding on the uninfected breast until the let-down occurs, then switch to the infected breast and breastfeed only until the breast is well-drained. If necessary, pump or hand express to soften the breast and relieve fullness.

• Put warm packs or ice packs on the infected area to relieve pain. Warm washcloths, a warm shower or tub bath or soaking the breasts in a pan of warm water works well. Some women prefer cold packs and use bags of frozen peas wrapped in a cold washcloth.

• Drink enough fluid to satisfy your thirst. Water and unsweetened fruit juices are suggested.

• Take acetaminophen or ibuprofen for pain.

• Get plenty of rest. Take the baby to bed with you to save time and energy.

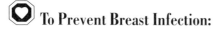 **To Prevent Breast Infection:**

• Position the baby correctly on the breast.

• If you delay or miss a feeding or if the baby breastfeeds poorly, hand express or pump to soften the breast and relieve fullness.

• Use 2-3 different breastfeeding positions each day.

• Do not delay or miss feedings.

• Avoid bras that are too tight or bind, making it difficult to relieve fullness in all parts of the breast. Avoid bras with underwires.

• Wean gradually. Pump or hand express to relieve fullness.

Engorgement

 Cause:

Milk production begins 1-5 days after delivery, depending upon which baby this is for the mother. The fluids necessary for milk production are carried to the breast through the blood and lymph system. This increased supply of fluid collects in the breast tissue causing the breasts to swell. Early, frequent breastfeedings will relieve the swelling and soften the breasts. When breastfeedings are infrequent, delayed or missed, engorgement occurs. The breasts may be swollen, hard and painful. The skin may be thin, shiny and hot.

Recommended Treatment:

- Put ice packs on your breasts between breastfeedings. Bags of frozen peas wrapped in a wet washcloth work well.*

- Hand express or pump a small amount of milk or colostrum to soften the breast and position the baby correctly (see "Hand Expression," p.78). A warm shower or tub bath or soaking the breasts in a pan of warm water may make milk expression easier. However, heat will increase swelling, so you may need to limit the use of heat.

- Breastfeed every 1½-3 hours during the day and every 2-3 hours at night. To increase the flow of milk, gently massage the breast in a circular pattern while the baby is breastfeeding, using the flat part of your hand (Illustration 14). If your breasts are still full, hand express or pump to relieve fullness.

- Wear a bra for comfort and support. Avoid bras that are too tight or bind, making it difficult to relieve fullness and soften the breasts. Avoid bras with underwires.

- Do not use a nipple shield. It decreases nipple stimulation, milk production and milk release.

*Some women choose to use cold, raw, cabbage leaves on the breasts after each feeding to relieve engorgement. Why cabbage leaves relieve engorgement is unclear. There may be a substance in the leaves which decreases swelling or it may be the temperature of the leaves.[29,30] Rinse the leaves well in cold water before use. Place the leaves on the breasts with the nipples exposed until the leaves wilt (15-20 minutes).

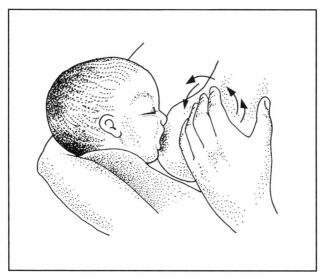

ILLUSTRATION 14: Use breast massage to relieve fullness and encourage the flow of milk.

To Prevent Engorgement:

• Breastfeed as soon as possible after birth.

• Breastfeed every 1½-3 hours during the day and every 2-3 hours at night.

• Breastfeed as long as the baby wishes on the first breast before offering the second breast.

• Offer both breasts at every feeding.

• Begin each breastfeeding on the breast offered last.

• If you delay or miss a breastfeeding or the baby breastfeeds poorly, hand express or pump to relieve fullness.

Leaking

 Cause:

Leaking often occurs during the early weeks when the baby is breastfeeding at irregular times. It may take 6-12 weeks for your baby to obtain a regular feeding schedule. Until that time, your milk supply will continue to change. While leaking is normal, it may not occur in every mother. Leaking can occur when you think about your baby, when you hear your baby or another baby cry, when you delay or miss a feeding and your breasts overfill or when you are making love and have an orgasm.

 Recommended Treatment:

• To control leaking, press firmly against the nipple of each breast with the palm of your hand or your wrist or fold your arms tightly across your chest.

• Nursing pads provide short-term protection and come in all shapes and sizes, disposable as well as reusable. You can even make your own pads using cloth diapers, cotton fabric or men's handkerchiefs. Change pads frequently. Do not use pads with waterproof liners.

• Choose clothing with light colors and small prints that will cover up a "multitute of mishaps."

• Breastfeed the baby before making love or going to bed. This will limit the amount of milk in the breasts and allow time for sex or sleep.

Plugged Duct

 Cause:

The narrow passages or ducts that carry newly-produced milk from the milk-producing cells to the collecting pools can become blocked. When breastfeedings are delayed or missed or when the baby breastfeeds poorly, milk can collect in the ducts and form a thick plug or a small lump. The area may or may not be painful.

Recommended Treatment:

- Put warm water on the plugged area before each feeding.
- Breastfeed more often during the day.
- Begin each feeding on the breast with the plug.
- Adjust the position of the baby's mouth on the breast (baby's nose or chin pointing toward the plug) to help remove the plug.
- Gently massage the plugged area while the baby is breastfeeding (Illustration 14).
- Pump or hand express after each breastfeeding to help remove the plug and relieve the fullness.
- Breastfeed in a position that will best relieve the fullness in the plugged portion of the breast.

To Prevent Plugged Ducts:

- Position the baby correctly on the breast.
- Use 2-3 different breastfeeding positions each day.
- Do not delay or miss feedings.
- If necessary, pump or hand express to relieve fullness.
- Avoid bras that are too tight or bind making it difficult to relieve fullness in all parts of the breast. Avoid bras with underwires.

Tender Nipples

 Cause:

Many mothers experience nipple tenderness or pain during the first few days of breastfeeding. Tenderness usually occurs at the beginning of a breastfeeding when the baby first "latches on" to the breast and draws the nipple into his mouth. If the baby is positioned correctly on the breast, the tenderness will only last a few seconds. If the pain continues throughout the feeding, you will need to recheck the baby's position carefully.

 Recommended Treatment:

• Put warm packs on the tender breast before each breastfeeding. A warm washcloth, a warm shower or tub bath or soaking the breast in a pan of warm water works well. After each breastfeeding use cold packs for pain relief. A bag of frozen peas wrapped in a wet washcloth works well.

• Position the baby correctly on the breast (Illustration 12). Lie the baby on his side facing your breast at the level of your chest. Tickle his upper and lower lip with your nipple until his mouth opens wide. Center your nipple in his open mouth and quickly bring him toward the breast (do not let him "nibble his way on"). His tongue should be over his lower gum, between his lower lip and the breast. His lips should turn out, like a fish, and lie flat against the breast. His chin should press firmly into the breast. His nose should gently touch the breast.

• If necessary express a small amount of milk or colostrum to soften the breast and position the baby correctly.

• Breastfeed on the least tender side first. When a let-down occurs switch to the tender side to relieve fullness in that breast. If both breasts are tender, soak the breasts in a pan of warm water and gently massage the breasts to encourage a let-down.

• If necessary, limit the breastfeeding time on the tender breast to 10-20 minutes and breastfeed more often, every $1\frac{1}{2}$-3 hours.

• Hold the baby close to prevent unnecessary pulling on the breast. Remember to break the suction before removing the baby from the breast.

- After each breastfeeding, put a small amount of colostrum or expressed breastmilk on the areola and nipple of each breast. Air dry nipples after each breastfeeding or gently blot the breast dry with a soft cloth. Brisk rubbing with a towel or washcloth will increase tenderness.

- Do not wash the nipples before each breastfeeding. Even water, used often, will dry the skin. Avoid soaps, creams and oils. If the nipples crack or bleed you can put a small amount of modified lanolin on the tender areas after each breastfeeding to provide relief and promote healing.[31]

- Should pain, cracking or bleeding continue, you might want to stop breastfeeding for 24 hours to let the nipple(s) heal. During this time you will need to pump or hand express to relieve fullness.

- If necessary, take acetaminophen or ibuprofen for pain. Take the medication 15 minutes before breastfeeding to provide pain relief while breastfeeding yet limit the effect of the medication on the baby.

To Prevent Tender Nipples:

- Follow postpartum breast and nipple care suggestions on p.31.

- Position the baby correctly on the breast, if necessary hand express to relieve fullness.

- Breastfeed as long as the baby wishes on the first breast before offering the second breast.

- Begin each breastfeeding on the breast offered last.

- Breastfeed every $1\frac{1}{2}$-3 hours during the day and every 2-3 hours at night.

- Use 2-3 different breastfeeding positions each day.

- Break the suction before removing the baby from the breast.

Yeast-like Fungus Infection (Thrush, Candidiasis, Moniliasis)

 Cause:

Candida or monilia is a yeast-like fungus that grows in dark, damp places. It can infect the birth canal, nipple and breast of the breastfeeding mother as well as the mouth and diaper-area of the baby. Candida is found in the birth canal (vagina) of most women, as a result, a baby can become infected during vaginal birth. Signs of infection appear 2-4 weeks after birth and include small, white patches in the mouth (Thrush) and a bright, red rash in the diaper-area. The infection is not serious however it can be very painful. Occasionally a baby will refuse to breastfeed.

The mother can become infected while breastfeeding. Signs of infection include small, red or white patches on the breast, red or purple nipples and sharp, shooting pain in the breast. Frequently the breasts look normal and severe pain is the only symptom. Some women have a thick, white, vaginal discharge with redness, itching and burning in the birth canal (vagina) as well.

Candidiasis can spread easily from one family member to another through close, intimate contact. Your partner can become infected during sex. Signs of infection include a red rash on or around the penis and small, white patches in the mouth.

Recommended Treatment:

- To prevent reinfection treat the mother and the baby. You may need to call your doctor as well as your baby's doctor. Treat your partner if signs of infection are present.

Mother: Rinse the breasts with clear water after each breastfeeding. Your doctor will recommend one of the following medications, Nystatin (Mycostatin) or Clotrimazole (Lotrimin). Put the cream or lotion on the nipple and areola of both breasts after each breastfeeding for 14 days. If the pain is severe, use one of the above medications with cortisone (Mycolog, Lotrisone) for the first 1-3 days. Gently massage the medication into the nipples.

Baby: Rinse the mouth with clear water after each breastfeeding. Your baby's doctor will prescribe a medication in solution form for the mouth and/or in cream or lotion form for the diaper-area. Apply the solution to the inside of the cheeks after each feeding. Use a clean, cotton swab for each cheek. Apply the cream or lotion to the red rash in the diaper-area during each diaper change.

• Expose your breasts as well as the baby's bottom to air and sunlight as often as possible. Be careful to avoid sunburn.

• Change nursing pads and diapers frequently. Do not use pads with plastic liners.

• Boil all rubber nipples and pacifiers daily for 20 minutes. Replace with new ones after the first and second week of treatment.

• Wash bras in hot, soapy water each day and rinse well. Boil all pump parts for 20 minutes each day.

• Wash your hands carefully before each breastfeeding and after each diaper change.

• Use condoms during sex. Do not let your partner's mouth come into contact with your breasts.

• Repeated infections may require 4-6 weeks of treatment. If necessary, choose a different cream or lotion as one may be more effective than another.

• Resistant infections that do not respond to the creams or lotions can be treated with pills or tablets taken by mouth. You will need to call your doctor for a prescription. In addition, you might want to avoid those foods that support the growth of fungus, such as alcohol, sugar, dairy products, wheat, nuts, peanut butter, dried fruits and fruit juices.[32]

⬡ To Prevent Yeast-like Fungus Infections:

• Wash your hands carefully before each breastfeeding and after each diaper change.

• Expose your breasts and the baby's bottom to air and sunlight whenever possible. Be careful to avoid sunburn.

• Change nursing pads and diapers frequently. Do not use pads with plastic liners.

• Avoid the use of nipple creams and lotions which may encourage the growth of yeast-like fungus or bacteria.

• Air dry nipples after each breastfeeding whenever possible.

SPECIAL SITUATIONS

Breastfeeding after Cesarean Birth

Cesarean birth is the surgical removal of the baby through an incision or opening made in the mother's abdomen. Nearly 20-30% of all births are cesarean births. Cesarean births are seldom planned, as a result, parents may experience many feelings including anger, relief, frustration, joy and sadness. Discuss your feelings openly with your doctor, family or friends. It may help to talk with other parents who have had an unplanned cesarean birth. While cesarean birth will not affect your ability to produce milk, pain and weakness may make it necessary to depend upon others for help. If mother or baby need special care, the start of breastfeeding may be delayed.

In the Hospital:

• Breastfeed as soon as possible after birth. If the start of breastfeeding is delayed for more than 24-48 hours, begin expressing your milk. Hand express or pump every 2-4 hours during the day and every 4-6 hours at night. Express each breast for 10-15 minutes, switching breasts every 5 minutes. An electric breast pump with a double collection set-up that lets you pump both breasts at the same time works best.

• Choose a comfortable position (Illustrations 9 & 10). Use extra pillows to protect the incision and provide support.

• Position the baby correctly on the breast (see "Beginning to Breastfeed," p.32, for step-by-step suggestions). You may need help with positioning, turning and burping (babies born by cesarean birth often have more mucus).

• Breastfeed on demand whenever the baby seems fussy or hungry. Expect to breastfeed every 1 $1/2$ - 3 hours during the day and every 2-3 hours at night. Breastfeed as long as the baby wishes on the first breast before offering the second breast.

• To promote healing and speed recovery:

　　✓ Increase the amount of protein (meat, fish, milk, eggs) and fiber (whole grains, raw vegetables) in your diet.

　　✓ Drink to satisfy your thirst (approximately 8-10 glasses a day), warm liquids increase bowel and bladder activity.

✓ Take short, frequent walks, mild exercise increases bowel activity and helps mothers regain their strength.

✓ Get plenty of rest, limit phone calls and visitors.

• Pain medication may be necessary for several days. Your doctor will order medication that is safe for breastfeeding mothers and babies. To provide pain relief yet limit the effect of the medication on the baby, take the medication 15 minutes before you breastfeed.

At Home:

• Breastfeed on demand or request whenever the baby seems fussy or hungry. Expect to breastfeed every 1½-3 hours during the day and every 2-3 hours at night. While demand or request feeding is recommended, some babies will not demand or ask to eat often enough or feed long enough to support rapid growth. Therefore, during the first 2-4 weeks, if your baby does not actively wake or cry, you may need to watch him for signs of lighter sleep such as sucking movements, sucking sounds or restlessness and offer the breast at those times.

• Keep the baby in the room with you to save time and energy.

• Get plenty of rest. Nap when the baby naps.

• Limit your activity. Avoid heavy lifting, household chores and brisk exercise for 4-6 weeks.

• To promote healing and speed recovery, continue:

   ✓ high protein, high fiber diet

   ✓ liquids to satisfy your thirst

   ✓ mild to moderate exercise

Breastfeeding the Premature Baby

The birth of a tiny baby born weeks or months premature can be scary. Why did this happen? Was it something I did? Was it something I didn't do? Will he live? Will he be normal? How long will he be in the hospital? Can I hold him? Can I breastfeed?

Premature babies can be breastfed, even those needing special care. Breastfeeding gives parents a chance to participate in the care of their baby, to do something that no one else can do, to parent in a very special way. Preterm mother's milk contains just the right amount of nutrients to meet a premature baby's needs. In addition, human milk contains special cells that protect babies against infections, which are common in premature babies.[33]

Let your baby's doctor know as soon as possible that you plan to breastfeed. The hospital staff can give you information on milk production as well as expression, collection and storage of breastmilk. In addition, they can you put in touch with other parents who have breastfed premature babies. These parents, along with the medical team, can help you develop realistic goals and provide you with much needed encouragement and support.

Early Feedings

Your baby may be too small or too sick to breastfeed in the beginning and will need to be fed a special liquid through a small tube or needle that is placed in one of his veins (intravenous feeding). As his condition improves, he will be fed your breastmilk through a small tube that is passed through his nose and into his stomach (gavage feeding).

Pumping

You should begin pumping as soon as possible after birth if your condition permits, within 24-48 hours. You will need to pump every 2-4 hours during the day and every 4-6 hours at night when awake. If you are pumping one breast at a time, pump each breast for 10-15 minutes, switching to the opposite breast every 5 minutes or when the flow of colostrum or milk slows down. An electric breast pump with a double collection set-up that lets you pump both breasts at the same time works best and saves time. In addition, double-pumping increases prolactin levels which increases milk production. Electric breast pumps are available for use while you are in the hospital. When you go home you can rent an electric breast pump from drugstores, medical supply companies, hospitals or private rental stations. Check with your baby's doctor or nurse for the location nearest you. Expressed colostrum or breastmilk can be collected and fed to your baby or frozen and used at a later date.

Your first attempts at pumping may only produce enough milk or colostrum to cover the bottom of the collection container. Don't get discouraged. It may take several days or weeks for you to see an increase in the amount of milk obtained. Like breastfeeding, pumping is a learned art. The following suggestions will increase the quantity of breastmilk obtained:

• Establish a routine, same time, same place. Choose a quiet comfortable place where you will not be disturbed. If necessary, take the telephone off the hook.

• Get organized, gather all of your supplies together as well as a healthy snack for mom.

• Wash your hands with soap and water and rinse well.

• Relax and think about your baby. Listening to a relaxation tape before pumping, making a phone call to the nursery to check on your baby's condition, looking at a picture of your baby or if possible sitting next to your baby's crib when you pump will increase the amount of milk obtained.[34]

• Put warm water on the breasts for 3-5 minutes. Warm washcloths (cover the cloths with plastic wrap to hold in the heat), a warm tub bath or shower or soaking the breasts in a pan of warm water works well.

- Gently massage the breasts in a circular pattern for 1-3 minutes using the flat part of your hand (Illustration 14).

- Tickle your nipples with your fingers to stimulate the let-down reflex.

- Moisten the pump flanges with water and center your nipples in the openings.

- With the pump on the lowest suction setting, pump until the flow of milk slows down (5-10 minutes), rest 3-5 minutes and repeat. If necessary, increase the suction as long as you stay comfortable.

Put the expressed milk into sterile containers provided by the nursery. Glass or hard plastic containers with solid lids are recommended. Label with your baby's name, your name, date and time and refrigerate immediately. Breastmilk can be stored in the refrigerator for 48 hours or in the freezer compartment of your refrigerator/freezer for 3 months (Illustration 15).[35,36,37] Store in single feeding portions to prevent waste.

Breastmilk storage recommendations for babies in the hospital:

Breastmilk	Room Temperature	Refrigerator	Refrigerator/ Freezer	Freezer
Fresh	Refrigerate immediately	48 hours	3 months	3 months
Defrosted in refrigerator	Use immediately or refrigerate	24 hours	Do not refreeze	Do not refreeze
Defrosted in pan of warm water	Use immediately	Do not save	Do not refreeze	Do not refreeze
Left in feeding container after feeding	Do not save	Do not save	Do not refreeze	Do not refreeze

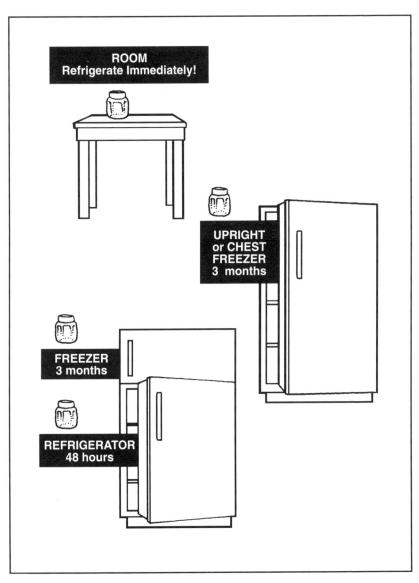

ILLUSTRATION 15: Breastmilk storage recommendations for sick or premature babies.

Getting to Know Your Baby as His/Her Condition Improves

As soon as your baby is able to leave the isolette for a period of time, place him underneath your clothing and cuddle him skin-to-skin against your chest (kangaroo care).[38] This early contact gives mothers and fathers a chance to care for their baby and to gain confidence in their ability to parent. Safe and secure against your chest, your body provides all the warmth your baby needs as he gets to know you. Many babies who participate in kangaroo care leave incubators sooner, gain weight faster and go home earlier. In addition, mothers who participate in kangaroo care often breastfeed for longer periods of time.

Beginning to Breastfeed a Sick or Premature Baby

Discuss your baby's readiness to breastfeed with the medical staff. While weight, gestational age and ability to bottle-feed are common guidelines, recent studies suggest that a baby's ability to suckle, swallow and breathe in an organized manner is a better indication of readiness to breastfeed and may appear at an earlier age.[39]

Once breastfeeding begins, remember that a premature baby will breastfeed frequently, every 1-2 hours, and tire quickly, so you will need to work at keeping him awake. Express a few drops of breastmilk onto the nipple and areola. Gently massage the breast while he is breastfeeding to increase the flow of hindmilk and the number of calories obtained at each feeding.[40,41] The football hold (Illustration 9A) may make it easier for you to keep the baby in a gently-flexed posture (C-shape). The Dancer's Hand position is helpful for tiny babies with weak muscles. Using your thumb and first finger to form a U-shape, support your baby's chin on the breast with your hand (Illustration 16).[42] Remember that these first breastfeedings are a learning experience for both of you, so relax and enjoy each moment.

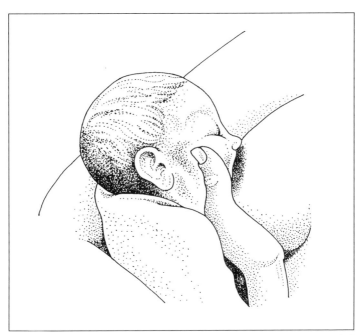

ILLUSTRATION 16: The dancer's hand position is helpful for tiny babies with weak muscles.

Providing a Supplement

Your milk supply may be low despite regular pumping and breastmilk or formula supplements may be necessary. To avoid nipple confusion, supplements can be given by teaspoon, medicine dropper, hollow-handled medicine spoon, cup, peridontal syringe or supplemental feeding device (Illustration 17).[43]

A supplemental feeding device is a plastic container filled with breastmilk or formula which hangs on a cord around the mother's neck. Two, thin pieces of plastic tubing stretch from the top of the container to the nipple of both breasts, where the tubing is taped into place. When the baby breastfeeds, he receives milk from the breast and supplement from the container. Once the baby is breastfeeding well and a good milk supply is established the supplement can be discontinued. If milk production remains low, medication (metoclopramide) can be prescribed to increase prolactin levels.[44,45]

As the condition of your baby improves and your confidence in your ability to care for your baby grows, you will be glad you chose to breastfeed. While breastfeeding a healthy, fullterm infant can be a challenge, breastfeeding a premature baby can seem overwhelming at times. However, the bigger the challenge, the greater the rewards.

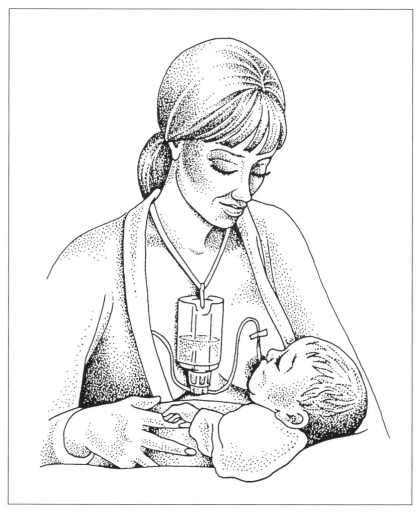

ILLUSTRATION 17: You can supplement a baby at the breast using a supplemental feeding device.

Breastfeeding Twins

You can produce enough milk to totally meet the nutritional needs of two (or more) babies. An understanding of the nature of milk production, "supply and demand", will be helpful. Nipple stimulation, produced by infant breastfeeding or milk expression is the stimulus for milk production. The more infant breastfeeding or milk expression which takes place, the more milk you will produce. Early, frequent breastfeedings or milk expression, if both babies need special care, will usually produce enough milk to meet the nutritional needs of two (or more) babies and help you get off to the best possible start. All the advantages of breastfeeding for mothers are multiplied when breastfeeding twins, especially the enforced skin-to-skin contact that will help you get to know each infant as an individual.

Planning Ahead

Be prepared to begin breastfeeding under many different circumstances, since cesarean birth, prematurity and other conditions resulting in the need for special care for one or both babies are more common with multiple births. Plan to attend childbirth preparation and cesarean birth classes early in your pregnancy, beginning in your fourth or fifth month. Share and discuss information about breastfeeding multiples with your partner. Locate resources for buying or renting a breast pump should milk expression be necessary. Contact LaLeche League and/or Mother of Twins Club and ask if they can put you in touch with a mother who has successfully breastfed twins. Choose a pediatrician who is knowledgeable about breastfeeding and believes that twins can be successfully breastfed. The encouragement and support of your partner, another breastfeeding mother of twins and your pediatrician will give you confidence in your abilities that is priceless.

Starting to Breastfeed

Ideally your babies' first breastfeeding will occur soon after delivery, within the first hour. While rooming-in or a modified version of it is possible with two babies, you may need to wait a day or two after a cesarean birth. Frequently breastfeedings are easier when babies are accessible and your confidence in handling them can grow while help is available. If rooming-in is not possible ask that both babies be brought to you for all breastfeedings. Remember that each twin is a single newborn needing 8-12 breastfeedings in a 24-hour period. If both infants require special care, begin expressing your milk 10-12 times a day within 24 hours after delivery.

The goal of frequent pumping is to stimulate prolactin release and establish milk production. Do not worry about the quantity of milk expressed. A regular pumping schedule will help to stimulate the release of oxytocin and condition the let-down reflex. When only one twin needs special care, pump one breast while the co-twin breastfeeds on the other breast to get maximum benefit of the let-down reflex. This will also increase the quantity of breastmilk obtained at a pumping session. The expressed breastmilk can then be stored and used at a later date for either twin.

Choosing a Breastfeeding Method

Almost any method of coordinating breastfeedings will work, as long as each twin breastfeeds 8-12 times in 24 hours. Many mothers breastfeed both babies on both breasts at every breastfeeding however you might want to breastfeed one baby on one breast at each breastfeeding. This will save considerable time especially if you breastfeed both babies at once.

To stimulate milk production in both breasts equally, your twins should take turns on the right and left sides. Some mothers alternate the breast each baby uses at every breastfeeding. It is less complicated however to rotate babies on a daily basis. If today Baby A breastfeeds on the right breast while Baby B breastfeeds on the left, then tomorrow Baby A will use the left breast and Baby B the right. Some mothers assign one particular breast to each baby for all breastfeedings, however, you may end up with two breasts that are two different sizes, due to differences in milk production based on the babies' individual needs. Also there are a few instances when one baby can't breastfeed for a brief period of time and the co-twin might be unwilling to breastfeed on both sides. If you do choose the "assign a breast" method, rotate breastfeeding positions so both eyes of each baby receive adequate exercise.

Simultaneous breastfeedings (at the same time) can simplify breastfeeding twins. Some mothers breastfeed twins simultaneously for all breastfeedings, some mothers never breastfeed simultaneously and others combine simultaneous and individual breastfeedings. Even if you find simultaneous breastfeedings difficult to master in the early months, you may want to try again at 3-4 months when most babies can readily latch on to the breast. Pillows become needed extra arms when placed under your arms and across your lap to prop, support and/or hold the babies in position.

The following simultaneous breastfeeding positions are the ones used most often (Illustration 18).

FOOTBALL HOLD: With the babies on their sides and their heads in each of your hands, tuck a baby under each arm. Use pillows for comfort and support. This position helps avoid pressure in the incision area after a cesarean birth.

CRISS-CROSS HOLD: With the babies' chests against your chest, cradle a baby in each arm, side-by-side. Use pillows for comfort and support. You might find this position more comfortable if your feet are propped on a stool or you sit in a recliner or you tailor-sit (Indian-style).

COMBINATION HOLD/LAYERED LOOK: Place Baby A in the traditional or cradle position. Place Baby B on a pillow at your side. Support Baby B's head in your hand and tuck his body under your arm. Gently "layer" the head of Baby B on top of the abdomen of Baby A. This position permits discreet breastfeeding and is especially helpful when one or more baby has difficulty latching on.

Two babies, each having as many needs as any single-born infant will mean more work no matter how you choose to feed them. This is important to remember on those days when you are sure you have competed in a breastfeeding marathon and you wonder if you will ever experience the "joys" of breastfeeding. (Of course the babies enjoy the benefits of breastfeeding from the very beginning.) By accepting all offers of help, surrounding yourself with a network of supportive people to boost your self-confidence and employing your sense of humor to maintain perspective, you will soon be numbering yourself among the mothers who have successfully breastfed multiples.

*For more detailed information you can obtain the booklets, *Mothering Multiples: Breastfeeding and Caring for Twins and Breastfeeding Twins, Triplets and Quadruplets*, by contacting Double Talk, P.O. Box 412, Amelia, Ohio 45102.

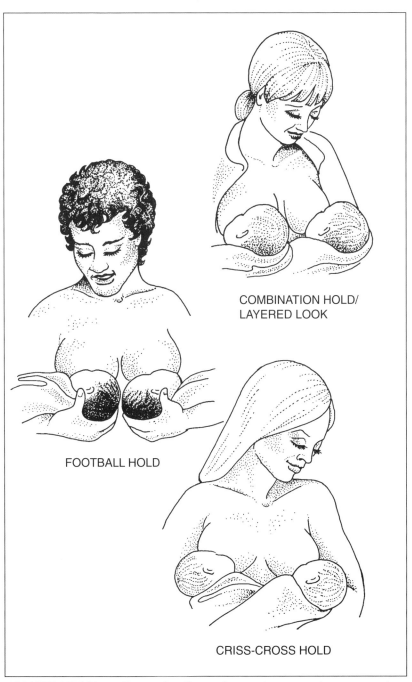

COMBINATION HOLD/
LAYERED LOOK

FOOTBALL HOLD

CRISS-CROSS HOLD

ILLUSTRATION 18: Breastfeeding twins at the same time saves time and energy.

Breastfeeding the Baby with Jaundice

Jaundice in the newborn is a common, complex and poorly understood problem. As a result, management of the jaundiced baby can be confusing, causing much concern for parents.[46]

Jaundice occurs in 50% of full-term infants and 75% of premature infants. Red blood cells provide oxygen to the body. Hemoglobin is the oxygen-carrying substance found in red blood cells. Due to the low level of oxygen inside the uterus, infants need extra red blood cells to meet their oxygen needs. After delivery, these extra red blood cells are no longer needed so they are broken down. When red blood cells break down, hemoglobin is released into the bloodstream. Hemoglobin contains bilirubin. The liver changes the bilirubin and excretes it into the stool where it is then eliminated. Sometimes it is difficult for the immature, newborn liver to remove the large quantity of bilirubin which collects after birth, and jaundice occurs. The skin and the whites of the eyes appear yellow. In addition, the baby may be sleepy and feed poorly.

Neonatal jaundice occurs 2-3 days after birth and disappears within 7-10 days. Recent studies found no difference in the peak level of bilirubin between breast and bottle-fed babies, however, breastfeeding may cause bilirubin levels to remain elevated for longer periods of time.[47] While many doctors question the need to treat breastfed babies with neonatal jaundice, other doctors recommend water supplementation, phototherapy or stopping breastfeeding for a brief period of time.[48] Discuss the choices carefully with your baby's doctor in an effort to avoid unnecessary confusion.

Pathologic or breastmilk jaundice are other causes of jaundice in the newborn. Pathologic jaundice is caused by blood incompatibility or liver disease. Different from neonatal jaundice, pathologic jaundice is often visible within 24 hours after birth and the bilirubin level may rise quickly. Prompt, medical attention is necessary. Breastmilk jaundice occurs in only a small percentage of infants about 1 in 100-200. The cause of breastmilk jaundice is unclear. There may be a substance in the breastmilk of some women that affects liver function. Breastmilk jaundice appears 4-6 days after birth and bilirubin levels peak on the 10th-14th day. In rare cases, if the bilirubin level continues to rise after the 14th day, you may need to rotate breast and formula feeds for 24 hours or stop breastfeeding for 24 hours and pump or hand express.

Breastmilk jaundice should not be confused with breastfeeding jaundice. Breastfeeding jaundice occurs when babies are not breastfed often enough. Expect to breastfeed every $1\frac{1}{2}$-3 hours during the day and every 2-3 hours at night. Expect 8-12 breastfeedings in a 24-hour period.

Often it is easy to identify the cause of jaundice. Many times a medical examination is necessary.

Management:

• Breastfeed as soon as possible after birth. Colostrum is a natural laxative which helps remove meconium from the lower bowel. Meconium is a thick, black, tarry substance that contains bilirubin.

• Breastfeed on demand or request at least every 2-3 hours. This will increase your milk supply, stimulate bowel movements in your baby and encourage the passage of meconium. Expect 8-12 breastfeedings and 4-8 bowel movements in a 24-hour period.

• Your doctor may suggest water or formula supplements after each breastfeeding if your milk does not appear by the third or fourth day after birth. Recent studies show no difference in the level of bilirubin in supplemented and unsupplemented babies.[49,50] In addition, water or formula supplements mean fewer breastfeedings and therefore less milk. In contrast, if you increase the number of breastfeedings, your milk supply will increase, your baby will have more stools and the bilirubin level will fall. Discuss this fully with your baby's doctor.

• Sometimes jaundice is treated with phototherapy, a fluorescent light-treatment. When the baby is exposed to a fluorescent light source the bilirubin level goes down. For protection, a small mask is placed over the baby's eyes. Phototherapy will increase your baby's fluid needs, so remember to breastfeed frequently, every $1\frac{1}{2}$-3 hours. Babies with jaundice, especially those under the lights, may be difficult to wake (see suggestions for waking a sleepy baby, p.37, item 11).

• Jaundice which occurs after you leave the hospital should be reported to your baby's doctor.

Breastfeeding the Baby with a Family History of Allergic Disease

Parents who have a personal or family history of allergic disease such as asthma, hay fever, allergic rhinitis, chronic ear infections or eczema should seriously consider breastfeeding their babies.

Breastfeeding during the first year of life can reduce the occurrence of allergic symptoms (gas, diarrhea, vomiting, fussiness, skin rashes) and frequent upper respiratory infections in sensitive babies.[11] In addition, the development of food allergies is greatly increased by the early introduction of foods other than breastmilk.[10] Parents who have a strong personal or family history of allergic disease or who have had a previous child with allergic problems should consider breastmilk only, for the first 6 months, avoiding all formula and solid food supplements during this time.

When supplements are introduced, the new foods should be added one at a time at weekly intervals. By doing this, it will allow you to clearly identify those foods which produce allergic symptoms. Cow's milk, eggs, peanuts (peanut butter) and meats should be eliminated from the infant's diet for the first six months and restricted for the next six months. If formula supplements are necessary, avoid cow's milk-based formulas and choose soy-based formulas instead. If allergic symptoms occur and breastfeeding is not possible or breastmilk is not available, non-allergenic formulas can be recommended by your baby's doctor.

Occasionally allergic symptoms develop in exclusively breastfed babies. Food proteins can be found in breastmilk in small quantities. In extremely sensitive babies, these proteins may occur in large enough amounts to cause allergic symptoms. In an effort to identify the cause of the symptoms, the mother's diet will need to be restricted. Foods eaten by the mother that can cause reactions in the infant are cow's milk, eggs, nuts and wheat (Illustration 19). You will need to eliminate these foods from the mother's diet for three weeks, then re-introduce the foods one at a time leaving 5-7 days between. It is unlikely that all the foods are the cause of the symptoms. By re-introducing the foods one at a time, it should be possible to determine which food or foods is the cause. If the restricted diet does not improve the baby's symptoms, the mother's diet can be returned to normal immediately and the baby's doctor should be consulted.

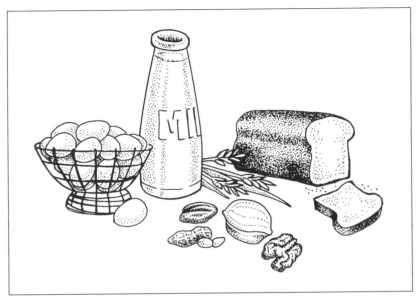

ILLUSTRATION 19: Foods eaten by the mother which may cause allergic symptoms in the baby.

Breastfeeding does not prevent allergic disease, but in many cases will delay the onset of symptoms for many years. This will allow the baby to mature and be better able to handle those symptoms that may develop in the future.

In severe cases, environmental control is recommended as well. Again, early exposure to tobacco smoke, heavy dust and animal dander can increase the risk of sensitivity and allergy.[9]

BREASTFEEDING AND THE WORKING MOTHER

Many mothers working outside the home continue to breastfeed. The special closeness which breastfeeding provides makes the separation of mother and baby and the return to work easier. Unfortunately, many mothers do not realize how easy it is to combine breastfeeding and working and stop breastfeeding when they return to work. The following suggestions will help you plan ahead so that the benefits of breastfeeding for mother and baby can continue.

Decide When You Will Return to Work

Whether you return to work after six weeks or six months will depend upon your own individual needs and circumstances. For many mothers the decision to return to work is not a choice but a necessity. While some mothers return to work full-time, others are able to arrange flexible part-time schedules that support breastfeeding. Many employers provide work options such as working out of the home, job sharing (sharing a full-time job with another person) and working part-time at the job location and part-time at home. Discuss these options with your employer as early in your pregnancy as possible.

Decide Who Will Take Care of Your Baby

Choosing childcare will be your most difficult task. While cost and convenience are necessary considerations, it is important that you choose someone you trust and someone who is supportive of breastfeeding. Childcare options include taking the baby with you to work, leaving the baby with an individual, either in your home or their home, taking the baby to a childcare center or arranging work schedules so that one parent is always available to care for the baby. If you plan to breastfeed your baby during working hours you might want to choose an individual or childcare center near your work place or arrange to have the baby brought to you for feedings.

Learn How to Express and Collect Breastmilk

Mothers who plan to supplement with breastmilk may begin expressing and collecting as soon as milk production begins. You can express from one breast while the baby breastfeeds from the opposite breast or you can express between feedings. Breastmilk can be stored at room temperature for 4 hours, in the refrigerator for 48 hours, in the freezer section of your refrigerator/freezer for 3 months and in an upright or chest freezer for 12 months (Illustration 21).[35,36,37]

Depending upon your baby's age and ability, you may choose to supplement with expressed breastmilk, solid food or infant formula. Your baby's doctor can recommend a specific formula. Occasionally babies react to non-breastmilk supplements, which may explain fussiness or a change in stool pattern. Regardless of your supplement choice, expression of breastmilk at least once during your working day may be necessary if you are going to be away from your baby for more than six hours. Breast fullness which is not relieved will cause your milk supply to decrease.

Your first attempts at milk expression may barely produce enough milk to cover the bottom of the collection container. Don't get discouraged. Much like the art of breastfeeding, success comes with practice.

Introduce a Supplement

Once your baby is breastfeeding well, about 4 weeks after birth, you can introduce an occasional supplement. Introducing a supplement too soon might confuse your baby's suckling pattern and decrease your milk supply. However, if your work schedule requires that you be away from your baby during feeding times, you need to know that he will accept food from something other than the breast. You can use a cup, medicine dropper, hollow-handled medicine spoon or bottle, whichever you prefer. Depending upon the baby's age and ability, you can supplement with expressed breastmilk, infant formula or solid food. Doctors frequently recommend breastfeeding alone for the first 4-6 months, then solid foods are slowly introduced, reducing the need for breastmilk. However, breastmilk or infant formula is necessary during the first year of life.

Babies sometimes refuse supplements offered by mother. Frequently a brother, sister, father or baby-sitter will be more successful. Should you choose to place the supplement in a bottle, try different nipple shapes and sizes until you find one that the baby will accept. Some mothers choose to avoid supplements altogether with "reverse-cycle" breastfeeding. "Reverse-cycle" breastfeeding means letting the baby sleep during the day while you are at work and breastfeeding in the evening and at night when you are together.

Guidelines for Returning to Work

- Avoid all supplements until your baby is breastfeeding well, about 4 weeks after birth. Use this time to increase your milk supply and learn to breastfeed.

- Practice expressing breastmilk from one breast while the baby breastfeeds from the opposite breast and between breastfeedings throughout the day. Collect, label and freeze in single feeding portions.

- Introduce an occasional supplement using expressed breastmilk or infant formula. You can put the supplement in a cup, medicine dropper, hollow-handled medicine spoon or bottle, whichever you prefer. Pump or hand express to relieve breast fullness.

- Continue to breastfeed and enjoy this time with your baby.

- Breastfeed before you go to work and as soon as you return. This will limit the amount of milk you will need to express while you are away and relieve fullness when you return. To make certain that your baby will be hungry when you return, ask the babysitter to avoid feeding the baby for 1-2 hours before.

- Pump or hand express while you are away to relieve fullness. Overfilling of the breasts is not only uncomfortable but may lead to plugged ducts, breast infections or a decrease in your milk supply over a period of time.

- Breastfeed more often when you and your baby are together to maintain your milk supply.

Regardless of how well you prepare for your return to work, there will still be a period of adjustment. Excitement, nervousness, guilt, sadness and joy are a few of the emotions you may experience. These feelings are normal. With time you will adjust priorities and establish routines and your confidence in your decision will grow. Support and encouragement from people around you is important, so don't hesitate to ask for help.

Any length of time you choose to breastfeed is wonderful. More important than how long you breastfeed or how often, is that it be an enjoyable experience for mother, father and baby.

COLLECTION/STORAGE OF BREASTMILK

Breastmilk can be collected by hand expression, hand pump, battery-operated pump or electric pump. Mothers who plan to pump infrequently will find that hand expression or a hand pump works well. Mothers who need to pump daily or for many weeks or months may choose to rent an electric pump. Mothers who choose to use a pump should still learn to hand express. Hand expression is economical and easy, something every breastfeeding mother should know.

Your first tries at expressing breastmilk may only produce enough milk to cover the bottom of the collection container. Donít get discouraged. It may take several days or weeks before you see an increase in the amount of milk obtained. Patience and practice are the keys to success. In the beginning you may want to express and collect from one breast while the baby nurses from the opposite breast. This will encourage a let-down and increase the flow of milk. As your confidence grows, you may want to express milk early in the morning and/or between breastfeedings when the breasts feel full. It is important that you relax, think about your baby and allow the milk to let-down. A warm shower or tub bath, warm washcloths or soaking the breasts in a pan of warm water along with breast massage and nipple stimulation may encourage a let-down and increase the flow of milk.

Hand Expression

• Choose a quiet, comfortable place.

• Wash your hands with soap and water and rinse well.

• Put warm water on the breasts for 3-5 minutes.

• Gently massage the breasts in a circular pattern for 1-3 minutes using the flat part of your hand (Illustration 20).

• Tickle your nipples with your fingers.

• Relax, think about your baby and allow the milk to let-down.

• Gently support the breast with one or both hands, thumb above and fingers below.

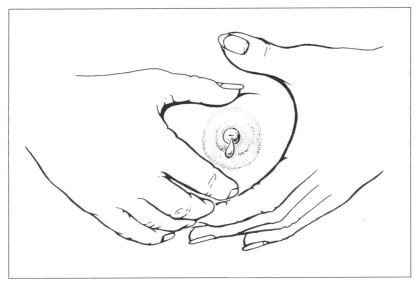

ILLUSTRATION 20: Hand expression makes removal of milk from the breast economical and easy.

- Place the thumb and first two fingers opposite each other just outside the edge of the areola, away from the nipple.

- Press in toward the chest, then slowly bring the thumb and fingers together, compressing the breast between the thumb and fingers. Do not squeeze or pinch. Do not compress the nipple itself.

- Change the position of the thumb and fingers on the breast and repeat the press, compress motion until all parts of the breast have been ex pressed and the flow of milk slows down (3-5 minutes). If your breast is the face of a clock position the thumb and fingers at 6 and 12, 1 and 7, 2 and 8, 3 and 9 etc.

- Repeat the procedure on the opposite breast. You will need to express each breast several times until the desired amount of milk has been collected or the breasts feel soft (20-30 minutes).

Expressing With a Breast Pump

- Wash your hands with soap and water and rinse well.

- Put warm water on the breasts for 3-5 minutes.

- Gently massage the breasts in a circular pattern for 1-3 minutes using the flat part of your hand.

- Tickle the nipples with your fingers.

- Relax, think about your baby and allow the milk to let-down.

- Moisten the pump flange(s) with water. Center your nipple(s) in the opening. Follow the directions which come with each pump.

- Wash the pump after each use in hot, soapy water and rinse well. During working hours, rinse with hot water and wash well when you get home.

The collection container which comes with many of the pumps can also be used for storage.

Choosing a Breast Pump

The following suggestions will help you choose the breast pump that is right for you:

- Factors to consider include: reason for use (to increase your milk supply, to establish a milk supply, to provide an occasional supplement, to nourish a preterm infant), frequency of use, effectiveness, ease of operation, ease of cleaning, availability, durability and cost.

- Features to consider include pressure range, suction control, flange size and shape, storage capacity and backflow protection.

- Mothers who plan to pump infrequently (once or twice a week) should consider hand expression, a hand pump or a battery-operated pump.

- Mothers who prefer to pump one breast while the baby breastfeeds from the opposite breast should consider a squeeze-handle hand pump, a battery-operated pump or a semi-automatic electric pump, all of which can be easily operated with one hand.

- Mothers who plan to pump frequently (one or more times a day) should consider an automatic electric pump with a built-in pressure cycle, similar to a breastfeeding baby.

- An automatic electric pump equipped with a double-collection system that allows you to pump both breasts at once, saves time and energy. In addition, double-pumping increases prolactin levels which increases milk production.

Your first tries at pumping milk may only produce enough milk to cover the bottom of the collection container. Don't get discouraged. It may take several days or several weeks before you see an increase in the amount of milk obtained. Like breastfeeding, pumping is a learned art.

Pumping technique is equally as important as your choice of pump. Try to establish a routine. Choose a quiet, comfortable place. Put warm water on your breasts for several minutes. Gently massage your breasts and tickle your nipples to encourage the flow of milk before you begin to pump. Relax and think about your baby. Looking at a picture of your baby, listening to music, listening to a relaxation tape or sitting near your baby when you pump, will increase the amount of milk obtained. Like breastfeeding, patience and practice are the keys to success.

Suggestions for Choosing a Breast Pump

Reasons for Use and/or Purchase	Hand Expression	Hand Pump	Battery Pump	Semi-Automatic Electric Pump	Automatic Electric Pump
To begin a milk supply					X
To increase a milk supply	X	X	X	X	X
To provide an occasional supplement	X	X	X	X	
To provide breastmilk for a hospitalized preterm infant					X
Mothers who plan to pump 1-2 times a week	X	X	X	X	
Mothers who plan to pump one or more times a day				X	X
Mothers who prefer to pump one breast while the baby breastfeeds from the opposite breast	X	X	X	X	
Mothers who prefer to double-pump				X	X

Storage

• Use a container with a wide opening, a mayonnaise or peanut butter jar works well. Wash in hot, soapy water and rinse well or clean in a dishwasher.

• Pour the expressed milk into a plastic or glass container for storage. Allow room for expansion if the milk is to be frozen.

• Label all containers with the time and date.

• Place a single serving in each container. More than one container can be defrosted if larger amounts are needed.

• Breastmilk can be stored at room temperature for 4 hours, in the refrigerator for 72 hours, in the freezer section of a refrigerator/freezer for 3 months or in an upright or chest freezer for 12 months (Illustration 21).[35,36,37]

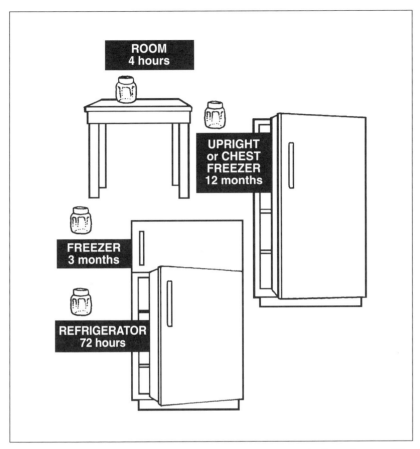

ILLUSTRATION 21: Breastmilk storage recommendations for healthy babies.

- Breastmilk stored in the freezer, should be placed in the middle of the freezer compartment. Do not store breastmilk on the freezer door.

- To defrost, place the unopened container in the refrigerator or in a pan of warm water. Do not defrost in a microwave. A microwave reduces the level of vitamin C, destroys live cells and heats the milk unevenly.[51]

- Serve breastmilk at room temperature. Heating destroys live cells and important nutrients.

• Breastmilk that has been defrosted in the refrigerator must be used within 24 hours.[37] Breastmilk that has been defrosted in a pan of warm water must be used within 4 hours.[37] Throw away any breastmilk left in the feeding container (bottle, cup etc.). Do not save for later use.

• You may combine several, small amounts of fresh breastmilk together to make one feeding or you can layer and combine fresh milk and frozen milk. However, you must chill the fresh milk in the refrigerator first to avoid defrosting the frozen layer.

Breastmilk storage recommendations for babies at home

Breastmilk	Room Temperature	Refrigerator	Refrigerator/ Freezer	Freezer
Fresh	4 hours	72 hours	3 months	12 months
Defrosted in refrigerator	4 hours	24 hours	Do not refreeze	Do not refreeze
Defrosted in pan of warm water	Use immediately or refrigerate	4 hours	Do not refreeze	Do not refreeze
Left in feeding container after feeding	Do not save	Do not save	Do not refreeze	Do not refreeze

WEANING

How long you breastfeed depends upon your own feelings and the needs of your baby. Some mothers choose to breastfeed for several weeks, several months or several years. Some babies lose interest in breastfeeding between six and twelve months when solid foods or a cup are introduced. Occasionally, circumstances occur which require the separation of mother and baby and make weaning necessary. More important than when you choose to wean or why, is that the process be slow. Weaning, particularly sudden weaning may cause feelings of sadness and guilt. This can be due to the sudden decrease in prolactin, as well as the unexpected end of the breastfeeding relationship. While these feelings are normal and will pass with time, it may help to talk about them.

Suggestions for Weaning Slowly

• Replace one breastfeeding at a time with solids or liquids depending on the baby's age and ability. Choose a breastfeeding in which the baby is least interested.

• Frequently babies refuse supplements offered by mother. You might want to ask a brother, sister or father to help with replacement feedings.

• Replace one breastfeeding every 3-5 days until weaning is complete.

• Increase cuddling time. Separation from the breast should not mean separation from mother.

• Distract an active and curious toddler with games, outdoor play and story-telling.

• Offer foods that are not available from the breast yet appeal to small children. Apple juice, grape juice, chocolate milk or finger foods are suggested.

• Expect some milk production to continue for 4-6 weeks.

• If sudden weaning is necessary, put ice on the breasts to relieve pain and reduce engorgement. Bags of frozen peas wrapped in a wet washcloth work well.

• Hand express or pump a small amount of milk to relieve fullness. A warm shower or tub bath may make milk expression easier.

COMMON QUESTIONS

Will breastfeeding change the size and shape of my breasts?

No. Breastfeeding does not permanently change breast size and shape. Many women who have had children notice that their breasts become smaller and sag or droop after birth. These changes are caused by pregnancy and are influenced by heredity, age and weight gain. Usually, the more weight you gain during pregnancy, the more your breasts will shrink or sag when the added pounds are lost. This is true whether you choose to breastfeed or bottle-feed.

Can I breastfeed and still lose weight?

Yes. Milk production requires 500-1000 calories each day. While you may add 500 extra calories to your diet and still lose weight, many mothers do not require additional calories to produce an adequate supply of milk. Fat deposited during pregnancy will usually satisfy your calorie needs. Frequently mothers find that "dieting" has never been easier and work, instead, to maintain their weight.

Must I follow a special diet?

No. As long as you eat a variety of foods from the basic food groups (breads, fruits, vegetables, dairy products, proteins and fats), drink to satisfy your thirst and continue your prenatal vitamins, both you and your baby should be fine. Occasionally certain foods in your diet will make your baby fussy. Milk products, nuts, eggs, chocolate, coffee or tea may be the cause. Should this happen you will need to limit that particular food.

What if I become ill and need medication?

Many medications are safe for breastfeeding mothers and babies. Check with your doctor before taking any medication. Make certain he knows that you are breastfeeding so that he can recommend medication that is effective yet safe.

Won't breastfeeding "tie me down"?

Yes and no. In the beginning, when babies are feeding frequently and irregularly, breastfeeding can be time-consuming. However, once your milk supply is well-established and the baby is feeding at regular times (about 6-12 weeks after birth) you will find it easier to come and go. If necessary a supplement can be given using expressed breastmilk or infant formula. You may use a cup, hollow-handled medicine spoon, medicine dropper, teaspoon or bottle, whichever you prefer.

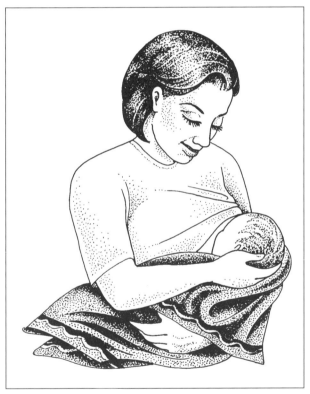

ILLUSTRATION 22: With a little practice, mothers can breastfeed discreetly anywhere.

I want to breastfeed but what if I find it embarrassing?

Some mothers feel embarrassed when they first start to breastfeed, others do not. How you feel will depend on your breastfeeding experience as well as the experience of those around you. Unfortunately, many people see the breast as a sexual object. As a result, many women are uncomfortable handling or exposing their breasts, even for something as natural and wonderful as breastfeeding. Be aware of your own feelings. If necessary, find a private place to breastfeed. Unplug the telephone. Put a small sign on your front door, "Hungry baby, do not disturb." With patience and practice your confidence in your decision to breastfeed will grow. Remember, experienced mothers can breastfeed discreetly and modestly anywhere (Illustration 22).

How can I tell if my baby is getting enough to eat?

The amount of milk taken from the breasts at each feeding cannot be measured, as a result, many mothers worry that their babies are getting enough to eat. Remember one important fact about your baby, "Nothing comes out the bottom unless something goes in the top." Two simple observations will help to reassure you:

• After the first 3 days, expect a minimum of 4 stools (bowel movements) a day for the next 6-12 weeks. Each stool will be yellow and watery with very little solid material and very little odor. The stool will look like sesame seeds and cottage cheese mixed with brown mustard. After the first 6-12 weeks, expect larger, softer, formed stools every 1-5 days.

• Expect 6-10 wet diapers in a 24-hour period. Most disposable diapers absorb liquid so well, it is difficult to tell if a baby is urinating frequently. However, a change in your baby's stool pattern is the first sign that he may not be getting enough to eat.

Do I need to give my baby vitamin and mineral supplements?

No. If you have a healthy, full-term infant, breastmilk provides all the vitamins (A, C, D and E) and minerals (iron and fluoride) he needs for the first six months of life. A daily dose of Vitamin D is recommended for those infants whose mothers are poorly nourished, or for those infants who are dark-skinned and get little sun exposure. Babies store enough iron in their liver during the last weeks of pregnancy to meet their iron needs for 6 month. After 6 months, iron-fortified cereal is recommended.

If I breastfeed, can I still give my baby a pacifier?

Yes and no. Once you have a good supply of milk and your baby is breastfeeding well, about 4 weeks after birth, you can offer a pacifier.[52] However, if you offer a pacifier too soon you can confuse your baby and limit your milk supply. In addition, pacifier use can increase the risk of ear infections and cause early weaning. Many breastfed babies prefer to suck on their fists, thumbs or fingers and refuse pacifiers.

If my baby has colic can I still breastfeed?

Yes. Colic, long periods of fussing and crying each day for no apparent reason, occurs in 10-20% of newborns. Colic occurs in formula-fed babies as well as breastfed babies. The symptoms usually appear 2-6 weeks after birth and disappear by 12-16 weeks of age. The cause of colic is unclear. Occasionally overfeeding or something in the infant's or the mother's diet can cause fussiness. Often no cause is found. If you have a fussy baby, offer one breast at each feeding. The result will be a low volume, low sugar, high fat meal rather than a high volume, high sugar, low fat meal. In addition, avoid cow's milk-based formulas in your baby's diet and milk products, eggs, nuts and wheat in your diet (see "Breastfeeding the Baby with a Family History of Allergic Disease," p.72).

Constant sounds or vibrations like a vacuum cleaner, clothes dryer, car engine or untuned television may soothe a fussy baby. A warm compress on the abdomen can also be effective. A warm tub bath, a warm washcloth or a warm hot water bottle works well. While colic seldom lasts more than 16 weeks, it can seem like 16 years! A mother unable to calm her baby feels guilty. A father unable to calm his partner feels helpless. If the fussiness continues, medication can be helpful. You will need to call your baby's doctor for a prescription.

Weaning is seldom necessary. Frequently, the use of infant formula makes the symptoms worse. As the infant grows and the gastrointestinal tract matures, the symptoms will improve. However, remember, a normal infant cries 2-3 hours a day.[53]

I tried to breastfeed my baby but I was unable to produce enough milk. How can I keep this from happening again?

Nearly every mother is capable of producing enough milk to nourish her baby. When a mother does not produce enough milk it is usually the result of too little information, incorrect information or too little support. The following suggestions will help you establish and maintain a good milk supply:

• Breastfeed on demand whenever the baby seems fussy or hungry. Expect to breastfeed every $1\frac{1}{2}$-3 hours during the day and every 2-3 hours at night. Occasionally a sleepy baby will not demand to eat often enough. Therefore, during the first 2-4 weeks, if your baby does not actively wake or cry to be fed, you may need to watch for signs of lighter sleep such as sucking movements, sucking sounds or restlessness and offer the breast at those times.

• Breastfeed as long as the baby wishes on the first breast before offering the second breast. If the baby falls asleep and breastfeeds poorly on the first breast, break the suction, burp him, wake him and put him back on the first breast.

• Offer both breasts at every breastfeeding. However, do not be concerned if the baby seems satisfied with one breast. Remember, each breast can provide a full meal. It is more important that he breastfeed well on one breast than that he feed on both breasts.

• Begin each feeding on the breast offered last.

• Avoid the use of water or formula supplements during the first 4 weeks. Supplements can confuse the baby's sucking pattern and interfere with breastmilk production.

• Drink to satisfy your thirst (8-10 glasses a day). Water and unsweetened fruit juices are suggested. It is not necessary to drink milk to make milk. Mothers who eat large amounts of milk or milk products often have fussy babies.

• Eat a balanced diet.

• Get plenty of rest. Nap when the baby naps.

• Should problems occur, get help from people you trust.

How much weight should my baby gain in the beginning?

Your baby may lose 5% of his birth weight during the first week and regain that weight during the second week. After the first or second week, your baby should gain 4-8 ounces a week. Occasionally, a baby will gain less, however, breastfeeding patterns and techniques should be carefully reviewed.

I plan to give my baby a supplement using expressed breastmilk. How much milk will I need to express for a feeding?

A healthy, full-term baby needs $2\frac{1}{2}$ ounces per pound per day. For example, a 10 pound baby would eat $2\frac{1}{2}$ x 10, or 25 ounces a day. If the baby breastfeeds every 3 hours, or 8 times a day and eats 25 ounces a day, then he takes about 3 ounces at each breastfeeding. To be on the safe side, express 4 ounces of breastmilk but store the milk in 2 ounce quantities to avoid waste.

Some mothers prefer to use infant formula and choose a soy-based formula rather that a cow's milk-based formula. Check with your baby's doctor for a recommendation.

Will breastfeeding affect my sex life?

Some mothers have less desire for sex due to tiredness, fear of pregnancy or fear of pain. Others find that breastfeeding, alone, provides enough touching and holding to satisfy their sexual needs. Still others are eager to have sex. Discuss your feelings openly with your partner.

Many breastfeeding mothers have some dryness in the vagina that may cause pain during intercourse. A water soluble lubricant such as K-Y Jelly may be helpful. Put a small amount around the opening of the vagina (birth canal) before having intercourse.

When you have sex, you can experience sexual excitement (orgasm). Sexual excitement causes the release of oxytocin. Oxytocin causes the release of milk from the breasts. To avoid leakage of milk from the breasts during intercourse, breastfeed the baby before making love.

If I breastfeed can I still get pregnant?

Yes and no. While natural child spacing can occur with unsupplemented, unrestricted breastfeeding, breastfeeding schedules or routines that delay or decrease breastfeedings can result in a return of fertility (ability to get pregnant). Ovulation (egg release) and menstruation (monthly bleeding) may not occur while you are breastfeeding, particularly during the first 6-12 weeks, however, many women resume ovulation and menstruation sometime during the breastfeeding period. Therefore, if pregnancy is not desired, a reliable method of birth control is suggested. Your choices include diaphragm, condom, intrauterine device, cervical cap, vaginal sponge or spermicidal cream or foam. Birth control pills that contain estrogen and progestin (combination pills) are not suggested, however, birth control pills, implants (Norplant) or hormone injections (Depo-Provera) that contain progestin only are safe. Discuss the choices with your doctor. Remember, ovulation can occur before menstruation, therefore, do not assume that you are "safe" or protected until your first menstrual period.

If I become pregnant can I still breastfeed?

Yes. It is possible to breastfeed throughout your pregnancy and to have two infants at the breast after birth. This is called "tandem nursing." However, you must eat a balanced diet which includes extra calories and get plenty of rest. To provide the calories necessary for the rapid growth that takes place in the first year of life remember to breastfeed the younger infant first.

Do I need to stop breastfeeding when the baby's teeth come in?

No. The arrival of teeth does not make weaning necessary. Each of my children cut their first tooth at three months of age yet were breastfed more than a year. Occasionally, toward the end of a feeding, when the baby is no longer hungry, biting can occur in a playful manner. Simply remove the baby from the breast with a firm "no." If the baby is still hungry offer the breast again. If the biting continues, remove the baby from the breast for several minutes. He will quickly learn that biting results in removal from the breast and the biting should stop.

How long should I breastfeed?

Until you or your baby decide that it is time to stop. This may be several weeks, several months or several years. Doctors recommend breastfeeding, alone, for the first 4-6 months, then solid foods are slowly introduced reducing the need for breastmilk. However, breastmilk or infant formula is necessary during the first year of life.[54] Many women choose to breastfeed until the baby can be weaned easily to a cup (12-24 months).

What are growth spurts?

Growth spurts or frequency days commonly occur around 3 weeks, 6 weeks, 3 months, and 6 months. However, they can occur at any time. Your baby may be fussy and restless and want to breastfeed all the time. Well-meaning but inexperienced friends and relatives may suggest that "your milk isn't rich enough," that "you're not making enough milk," that "solid foods or a formula supplement are necessary," or that "it is time to stop breastfeeding." After 2-3 days of frequent breastfeedings, your milk supply will catch up with the increased demand and the length and frequency of breastfeedings will decrease. Feeling confident in your ability to breastfeed your baby is very important. Seek advice from experienced friends or relatives or a board certified lactation consultant in your community.

What are nursing strikes

A nursing strike occurs when a baby suddenly refuses to breastfeed. It can last for several feedings or several days. Sometimes the cause is easily identified, such as teething, fever, ear infection, stuffy nose (cold), constipation or diarrhea. Occasionally, menstruation or something in your diet will change the taste of your milk. Deodorant, perfume or powder placed on the mother's skin may cause the strike. Frequently no cause is found. Until the strike ends, you will need to hand express or pump to reduce fullness and maintain your milk supply. Continue to offer the breast, however, do not insist if the baby refuses. Give expressed breastmilk by teaspoon, eye dropper, hollow-handled medicine spoon or cup until breastfeeding resumes. Be patient and relax. Give your baby undivided attention. Nursing strikes seldom lead to weaning. With time the baby will return to the breast.

Can I breastfeed if I am HIV positive?

The Center for Disease Control (CDC) and the United States Public Health Service recommend that women in the United States who test positive for HIV do not breastfeed. However, in developing countries where the risk of death during the first year of life from diarrhea and other infections is high, breastfeeding is encouraged, even among HIV positive women.

Can I breastfeed if I use drugs?

Women who are chemically dependent and actively abusing drugs should not breastfeed. However, recovering drug users who remain drug-free can breastfeed. Close follow-up is recommended for both the mother and the baby.[55]

Can I exercise if I am breastfeeding?

Yes. Moderate exercise does not affect the quantity of milk produced. However, exercise increases the level of lactic acid in the milk and gives the milk a sour taste. In addition, some babies may refuse to breastfeed because of the perspiration on the skin surface. If this occurs, rinse the breast(s) before you breastfeed, or breastfeed no sooner than $1\frac{1}{2}$ hours after exercising.[56]

I had breast surgery. Will I be able to breastfeed?

Yes and no. As long as the milk ducts, nerves and blood vessels are intact, breastfeeding is possible. The most common surgical procedures include breast augmentation (insertion of implants), breast reduction (removal of breast tissue), lumpectomy (removal of a breast lump) and mastectomy (removal of a breast).

Lumpectomy and breast augmentation seldom affect your ability to produce milk. Women who have had a mastectomy can usually nourish a baby at the remaining breast. However, they may need to breastfeed more often in the beginning to increase their milk supply. Women who have had breast reductions often find that milk production is limited. Frequently, when a large amount of breast tissue is removed, nipples are repositioned on the newly formed breasts, damaging milk ducts.

Can I breastfeed if I have silicone breast implants?

Yes, women with silicone breast implants as well as other implants can breastfeed as long as the implants are not leaking.

When should I call my baby's doctor?

Problems can occur during the early weeks when a mother and baby are learning to breastfeed. You can prevent serious problems if you know the early, warning signs that your baby may not be getting enough to eat. If your baby is less than 6 weeks of age and any of the following occur, call your baby's doctor:

• fewer than 2 bowel movements a day during the first 3 days or fewer than 4 bowel movements a day during the next 6 weeks

• fewer than 6 wet diapers a day

• fewer than 8 breastfeedings a day; each feeding lasting less than 15 minutes

• no sign of suckling and swallowing when feeding

• no sign of a let-down reflex

• your baby is either restless and irritable or listless and sleepy for long periods of time

• your baby is gaining less than 4-8 ounces a week

• your baby is below birth weight at two weeks of age

Conclusion

Breastfeeding is a wonderful part of parenting. A chance to hold, to touch, to know your baby from the first moment of birth. Breastmilk is nature's way of protecting and nourishing your baby.

During the early 1900's efforts were made to improve upon nature. A tremendous amount of time and money was spent developing breastmilk substitutes. Infant feeding became a science of mixing and measuring. Mothers, fathers and babies were separated at birth. Rules and routines were strictly enforced. Breastfeeding became the exception while bottle-feeding became the norm. Parents choosing to breastfeed and professionals choosing to recommend breastfeeding had to justify the use of human milk for human infants. Routine use of breastmilk substitutes became the world's largest experiment without controls.[57] As a result, there was a serious increase in infant infection and infant death.[58,59] The advantages of breastfeeding as well as the dangers of bottle-feeding were quite clear.

Today the World Health Organization and the United States Department of Health and Human Services are working together to promote breastfeeding worldwide.[60,61] Every effort is being made to identify the barriers which keep parents from beginning to breastfeed or continuing to breastfeed.[62] Too little information, incorrect information, too little support and early use of breastmilk substitutes are just a few examples. Barriers exist in the hospital as well as the workplace. Hospital routines and inflexible work schedules that separate mothers and babies and limit the length and frequency of breastfeedings make continuation of breastfeeding difficult.

Most parents today know that breastfeeding is the best choice for every baby. Now parents need to know that breastfeeding is the right choice for every parent as well; that breastfeeding can be flexible; that breastfeeding can be fun.

Enjoyment is the measure of success. A firm desire to breastfeed, a clear understanding of how to proceed and encouragement and support from people you trust will increase your enjoyment of breastfeeding and assure your success. While breastfeeding is the natural way to feed your baby, breastfeeding does not always come "naturally." It is a learned art which requires preparation, practice and encouragement. Your partner, grandmother, mother, friend, physician, nurse, childbirth educator and lactation consultant are good sources of support. So don't hesitate to ask for help. With practice and patience your confidence in your ability to breastfeed will grow.

Regardless of your feeding choice, parenting is a tremendous challenge. It is the most difficult job you will ever do with the least amount of preparation. You will work twenty-four hours a day, seven days a week, fifty-two weeks a year. Your salary will be a smile, a laugh, a hug, a first word, a first step, a first tooth and without hesitation you would do it all again. Parenting is a special joy. Cherish each moment.

While breastfeeding may not seem the right choice for every parent, it is the best choice for every baby.

FOOTNOTES

1. Newcomb, Polly A.et al: Lactation and a reduced risk of premenopausal breast cancer. *The New England Journal of Medicine* 330(2):82-87, 1993.

2. United Kingdom National Case-Control Study Group: Breast feeding and the risk of breast cancer in young women. *British Medical Journal* 307:17-20, 1993.

3. Klaus, M., Kennell, J: *Maternal-Infant Bonding.* St. Louis, C.V.Mosby Co., 1976.

4. Nutrition Committee of the Canadian Paediatric Society and the Committee on Nutrition: Breastfeeding. *Pediatrics* 62:591, 1978.

5. Garza, Cutberto, Schanler, Richard, Butte, Nancy and Motil, Kathleen: Special properties of human milk. *Clinics in Perinatology* 14(1): 11-32, 1987.

6. Cunningham, A., Jelliffe, D.B., Jelliffe, E.F.P: Breastfeeding and health in the 1980s: a global epidemiologic review. *Journal of Pediatrics* 118(5): 659-66, 1991.

7. Kovar, Mary Grace, Serdula Mary, Marks, Janes, Fraser, David: Review of the epidemiologic evidence for an association between infant feeding and infant health. *Pediatrics* (Supplement) 75:167, 1985.

8. Howie, Peter, Forsyth, J. Stewart, Ogston, Simon A., Clark, Ann and du V Florey, Charles: Protective effect of breast feeding against infection. *British Medical Journal* 300:11-16, 1990.

9. Ashad, S.H., Stevens M.and Hide D.W.: The effect of genetic and environmental factors on the prevalence of allergic disorders at the age of two years. *Clinical Experimental Allergy* 23:504-511, 1993.

10. Bardare, Maria, Vaccari, Antonia, Allievi, Elisabetta, Brunelli, L., Coco, Francesca, de Gaspari, G.C. and Flauto, U.: Influence of dietary manipulation on incidence of atopic disease in infants at risk. *Annals of Allergy* 71:366-371, 1993.

11. Bruno, G., Milita, O., Ferrara, M., Nisini, R., Cantani, A. and Businco, L.: Prevention of atopic diseases in high risk babies (Long Term Follow-Up). *Allergy Practice* 14:181-187, 1993.

12. Lucas, A., Morley, R., Cole, T.J., Lister, G. and Lesson-Payne C.: Breast milk and subsequent intelligence quotient in children born preterm. *The Lancet* 339:261-264, 1992.

13. Frederickson, D.D., Sorenson J.R., Biddle, A.K. et al: Relationship of sudden infant death syndrome to breastfeeding duration and intensity. *American Journal of Diseases in Children* 147:460, 1993.

14. Mitchell, E.A., Aley, P. and Eastwood, J.: The National Cot Death Prevention Programme in New Zealand. *Australian Journal of Public Health* 16:158, 1992.

15. Scragg, L.K., Mitchell, E.A., Tonkin S.L. et al: Evaluation of the cot death prevention programme in South Auckland. *New Zealand Journal of Medicine* 106:8, 1993.

16. Chao, Solan: The effect of lactation on ovulation and fertility. *Clinics in Perinatology* 14:39, 1987.

17. Hatcher, Robert A. et al: *Contraceptive Technology 1990-1992*. New York, Irving Publshers, Inc., 1990, p. 301.

18. Pinilla T, Birch LL: Help me make it through the night: Behavioral entrainment of breastfed infants' sleep patterns. *Pediatrics* 91:436, 1993.

19. Minchin, Maureen K.: Positioning for breastfeeding. *Birth* 16:2, 1989.

20. Lawrence, R.A.: *Breastfeeding a guide for the medical profession*. St. Louis, C.V.Mosby Co., 4th edition, 1994, p. 231.

21. Lawrence, R.A.: *Breastfeeding a guide for the medical profession*. St. Louis, C.V.Mosby Co., 4th edition, 1994, p. 228-230.

22. Alexander JM, Grant AM, Campbell MJ: Randomised controlled trial of breast shells and Hoffman's Exercises for inverted and non-protractile nipples. *British Medical Journal* 304:1030, 1990.

23. Hewat, R.J. and Ellis D.J.: A comparison of the effectiveness of two methods of nipple care. *Birth* 14:41, 1987.

24. Frantz, Kittie B.: Managing nipple problems. *Excerpta Medica* 1980.

25. Spangler, Amy and Hildebrandt, Evelyn: The effect of modified lanolin on nipple pain/damage during the first ten days of breastfeeding. *IJCE* 8(3):15-19, 1993.

26. Lawrence RA: Breastfeeding a guide for the medical profession, St. Louis, C.V. Mosby Co., 4th edition:233, 1994.

27. DeCarvalhi, M. et al: Effect of frequent breastfeeding on early milk production and infant weight gain. *Pediatrics* 72:307, 1983.

28. Woolridge, Michael W.: The physiology of suckling and milk transfer. Conference of the International Lactation Consultant Association, 1989.

29. Rosier W: Cool Cabbage Compresses. *Breastfeeding Review* 12:28, 1988.

30. Nikodem VC, Danzinger D, Gebka N et al: Do cabbage leaves prevent breast engorgement? A randomized, controlled study. *Birth* 20:61, 1993.

31. Sharp DA: Moist wound healing for sore or cracked nipples. *Breastfeeding Abstracts* 12(2):19, 1992.

32. Clay LS et al: Clinical Moniliasis, *Journal of Nurse-Midwifery* 35(6):377. 1990.

33. Lucas A, Cole TJ: Breastmilk and neonatal necrotising enterocolitis, *The Lancet* 336:1519, 1990.

34. Feher S, Berger L, Johnson J, Wilde J: Increasing breastmilk production for premature infants with a relaxation/imagery audiotape. *Pediatrics* 83(1):57, 1989.

35. Hamosh M et al: Breastfeeding and the Working Mother: Effect of Time and Temperature of Short-term Storage on Proteolysis, Lipolysis, and Bacterial Growth in Milk. Pediatrics 97(4):492, 1996.

36. Ajusi JD, Onyango FE, Mutanda LN, Wamola: Bacteriology of unheated expressed breastmilk stored at room temperature. *East African Medical Journal* June:381, 1989.

37. HMBANA: Recommendations for collection, storage, and handling of a mother's milk for her own infant in the hospital setting, 1993.

38. Anderson, GC: Current knowledge about skin-to-skin (kangaroo) care for preterm infants. *Journal Perinatology* 11:216, 1991.

39. Meier P, Anderson, GC: Responses of small preterm infants to bottle- and breast-feeding. *MCN* 12:97, 1987.

40. Stutte PC, Bowles BC, Morman G: The effects of breast massage on volume and fat content of human milk. *Genesis* 10(2):22, 1988.

41. Bowles, Betty Carlson: Alternate Massage in Breastfeeding. *Genesis* 9:6, 1987/1988.

42. Walker, Marsha and Driscoll, Jeanne: Breastfeeding your premature or special care baby/A practical guide for nursing the tiny baby. Weston, MA: Lactation Associates, 2nd edition (8), 1989.

43. Lawrence RA: Breastfeeding a guide for the medical profession, St. Louis, C.V. Mosby Co., 4th edition:398, 1994.

44. Ehrenkranz RA, Ackerman BA: Metoclopramide effect on faltering milk production by mothers of premature infants. *Pediatrics* 78(4):614, 1986.

45. Budd SC et al: Improved lactation with metoclopramide. *Clinical Pediatrics* January:53, 1993.

46. Brown, Linda P.: Breastfeeding and jaundice: Cause for concern?. NAACOG's Clinical Issues in Perinatal and Women's Health Nursing 3(4):613-619, 1992.

47. Kivahan, C. and James, E.J.P.: The natural history of neonatal jaundice. *Pediatrics* 74:364, 1984.

48. Martinez JC et al: Hyperbilirubinemia in the breast-fed newborn: A controlled trial of four interventions. *Pediatrics* 91(2):470, 1993.

49. DeCarvalhi, M., Hall, M. and Harvey, D.: Effects of water supplementa- tion on physiologic jaundice in breast-fed babies. *Arch. Dis. Child* 56:568, 1981.

50. Maisels, M.J. et al: Clinical and laboratory observations:: Breastfeeding, weight loss and jaundice. *The Journal of Pediatrics* 102:117, 1983.

51. Quan R, Yang C, Rubenstein S et al: Effects of microwave radiation on anti-infective factors in human milk. *Pediatrics* 89:667, 1992.

52. Barros FC et al: Use of Pacifiers is Associated With Decreased Breast- Feeding Duration. *Pediatrics* 95(4): 497, 1995.

53. St. James-Roberts I: Persistent infant crying. *Arch Diseases Childhood* 66:653, 1991.

54. Kretchmer, N.: Summary gastrointestinal and immunologic development. *Pediatrics* (Supplement) 75:187, 1985.

55. Wilton J: Breastfeeding and the Chemically Dependent Woman. *NAACOG'S Clinical Issues in Perinatal and Women's Health Nursing* 3(4): 667, 1992.

56. Wallace JP, Inbar G, Ernsthausen K: Infant acceptance of postexercise breastmilk. *Pediatrics* 89(6):1245, 1992.

57. World Health Organization: Contemporary pattens of breastfeeding, report of the WHO collaborative study on breastfeeding. Geneva, 1981, World Health Organization.

58. Victora, C.G., Smith, P.G and Vaughan, J.P. et al: Evidence for protection by breastfeeding against infant deaths from infectious diseases in Brazil. *Lancet* 2:319, 1987.

59. Cunningham, A.S.: Breastfeeding and health. *Pediatrics* 73:416, 1984.

60. Report of the Surgeon General's workshop on breastfeeding and human lactation. Publication no. HRS-D-MC 84-2, Department of Health and Human Services, 1984.

61. Followup report: The Surgeon General's workshop on breastfeeding and human lactation. Publication no HRS-D-MC 85-2, 1985.

62. Spisak, S. and Gross, S.S.: Second followup report: The Surgeon General's workshop on breastfeeding and human lactation. Washington, D.C.: National Center for Education in Maternal and Child Health, 1991.

INDEX

ABOUT THE AUTHOR

Amy Spangler is a mother, nurse, author, lecturer and recognized authority on the subject of breastfeeding. She holds a bachelor's degree in nursing from Ohio State University and a master's degree in maternal and infant health from the University of Florida.

Amy has been teaching parent education classes for twenty years. Currently, she is Parent Education Coordinator for a private Ob/Gyn practice where she teaches Breastfeeding, Prenatal Nutrition, Prenatal Exercise, Preparation for Labor and Birth and Early Pregnancy classes. She has worked as a labor and delivery nurse, as an office nurse and surgical assistant in a private practice, and as a clinical instructor in a college of nursing.

Amy is an International Board Certified Lactation Consultant and a member of the International Lactation Consultant Association, the International Childbirth Education Association, the Association of Women's Health, Obstetric, and Neonatal Nurses, as well as La Leche League International.

She lives in Atlanta with her husband Dennis, a private practice physician, and their two sons, Matthew and Adam.

Additional copies of this book
may be ordered by writing to:

Amy Spangler's
BREASTFEEDING, A Parent's Guide
P.O.Box 501046
Atlanta, Georgia 31150-1046

Telephone 770.913.9332
Fax 770.913.0822